Current Topics in Microbiology and Immunology

Volume 423

The review series *Current Topics in Microbiology and Immunology* provides a synthesis of the latest research findings in the areas of molecular immunology, bacteriology and virology. Each timely volume contains a wealth of information on the featured subject. This review series is designed to provide access to up-to-date, often previously unpublished information.
2018 Impact Factor: 3.153., 5-Year Impact Factor: 4.143

More information about this series at http://www.springer.com/series/82

Jeffrey V. Ravetch · Falk Nimmerjahn
Editors

Fc Mediated Activity of Antibodies

Structural and Functional Diversity

Responsible Series Editor: Rino Rappuoli

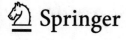 Springer

Editors
Jeffrey V. Ravetch
Department of Leonard Wagner Laboratory
of Molecular Genetics and Immunology
Rockefeller University
New York, NY, USA

Falk Nimmerjahn
Department of Biology
University of Erlangen-Nürnberg
Erlangen, Bayern, Germany

ISSN 0070-217X   ISSN 2196-9965   (electronic)
Current Topics in Microbiology and Immunology
ISBN 978-3-030-31055-4   ISBN 978-3-030-31053-0   (eBook)
https://doi.org/10.1007/978-3-030-31053-0

This Springer imprint is published by the registered company Springer Nature Switzerland AG
The registered company address is: Gewerbestrasse 11, 6330 Cham, Switzerland

Preface

If one looks through the lists of novel drugs targeting cancers, autoimmune/chronic inflammatory diseases, and infection, a molecule appearing very (if not most) frequently on that list will be antibodies of the Immunoglobulin G (IgG) isotype. Indeed, the much celebrated breakthrough in cancer immunotherapy is based on intact antibodies or antibody fragments, such as bispecific T cell engaging antibodies (BiTEs); and chimeric antigen receptors (CAR), which are antibody fragments expressed on T cells. Thus, antibodies are the new and old kid on the block for immunotherapy and surely will be in the focus of novel therapeutic approaches for many years to come. An in depth understanding of how antibodies mediate their activity is therefore of critical importance. Research of many groups over the last three decades has provided clear evidence that IgG binding to cellular Fc-receptors is essential for the activity of antibodies in vivo, emphasizing that the antibody constant region is much more than a framework carrying the variable domain, but rather is the essential—and actually not so constant—linker responsible for triggering IgG effector functions.

In autoimmunity, IgG antibodies play several important roles. Firstly, as autoantibodies they are drivers of autoimmune inflammation. Again, Fc-receptors have been identified as central players responsible for triggering the pro-inflammatory effects of autoantibodies. Second, IgG antibodies are used in the form of monoclonal antibodies targeting key pro-inflammatory cytokines or self-reactive immune cells. Finally, the infusion of polyclonal serum IgG preparations pooled from thousands of donors, also called intravenous IgG therapy (IVIg), is efficiently able to suppress a wide variety of chronic and acute autoimmune diseases, prompting many groups to investigate its mechanism of action and solve the mystery of IVIg activity. While many potential mechanisms of action of IVIg have been proposed over the years, one completely unexpected finding was that the sugar moiety attached to the IgG Fc-domain seemed to play a crucial role for the anti-inflammatory activity of these polyclonal IgG preparations. More in depth studies provided convincing evidence that especially IgG glycoforms carrying terminal sialic acid residues were responsible for the anti-inflammatory activity and that a family of type II Fc-receptors was involved in this anti-inflammatory pathway. A side effect of these observations was that it prompted many groups to re-visit the impact of glycosylation on immunoglobulin activity more broadly. This has led to the unexpected finding that not only IgG but also IgE antibody activity is regulated through glycosylation. Of note, especially one of the many sugar moieties attached to IgE was shown to be of critical importance for productive binding of IgE to its Fc-receptor. Coming to IgG and infection, IgG antibodies are essential to protect the host from infection or from the detrimental activity of bacterial toxins. Again, Fc-receptors were shown to be of major importance also for the activity of neutralizing antibodies, which were previously thought to mediate their activity independently of Fc-receptors. But antibodies are clearly not only beneficial in infection. Very recent studies have emphasized that glycovariants of virus specific IgG antibodies lacking fucose residues may be responsible for enhancing Dengue virus infection and pathology in hosts, also known as antibody dependent enhancement of infection. As IgG glycovariants lacking fucose modulate IgG binding to human FcgRIIIa (in humans) and FcgRIV (in mice), this again pinpoints towards an important role of Fc-receptors in this process. Finally, in a world of fading activity of antibiotics against bacteria more successful vaccination strategies will be of major importance. Harnessing the host through generating a most productive antibody response against microorganisms will be key to cope with this global threat. Using antibodies in combination with the antigens (that is: immune complexes) to boost immune responses is a very efficient and in fact the most natural way of enhancing immunity. Again Fc-receptors present on dendritic cells play a key role for such novel vaccination strategies.

In this book, we were able to bring together an exciting list of experts in the field covering all of these hot topics of antibody and Fc-receptor research. Stylianos Bournazos will look at Fc-receptors from an evolutionary point of view, while Graziano and Engelhardt will discuss the role of Fc-receptors for immunotherapy of cancer. The chapters of Beneduce and colleagues, Wang, and Shade and colleagues will discuss the importance of IgG glycosylation for the pro- and anti-inflammatory activities of IgG and IgE. Finally, the two chapters by Wen and Shi and Wieland and Ahmed will focus on how Fc-receptors impact vaccination and infection.

Naturally the examples mentioned above are only a fraction of the research, which is currently ongoing in the field of antibodies and Fc-receptors, but they clearly highlight how broad the impact of research on Fc-mediated activities of antibodies can be. We would like to thank all authors contributing to this volume again for their excellent contributions and we hope that it will stimulate new research ideas in this exciting area of immunology.

New York, USA   Jeffrey V. Ravetch
Erlangen, Germany   Falk Nimmerjahn

Contents

IgG Fc Receptors: Evolutionary Considerations

Stylianos Bournazos

Contents

Abstract Immunoglobulins (Ig), a critical component of the adaptive immune system, are present in all jawed vertebrates and through sophisticated diversification mechanisms are able to recognize antigens of almost infinite diversity. During mammalian evolution, IgG has emerged as the predominant Ig isotype that is elicited upon antigenic challenge, representing the most abundant isotype present in circulation. Along with the IgG molecule, a family of specialized receptors has evolved in mammalian species that specifically recognize the Fc domain of IgG. These receptors, termed Fcγ receptors (FcγRs), are expressed on the surface of effector leukocytes and upon crosslinking by the IgG Fc domain mediate diverse immunomodulatory processes with profound impact on several aspects of innate and adaptive immunity. FcγRs share a high degree of sequence homology among mammalian species and the ancestral locus, where the genes that encode for FcγRs are mapped, can be traced back early in mammalian evolution. FcγRs also share a number of common structural and functional properties among mammalian species and utilize highly conserved motifs for transducing signals upon engagement. Despite the high homology of FcγRs in diverse mammalian species, human FcγRs exhibit unique features relating to the gene organization, expression pattern in the

S. Bournazos (✉)
The Laboratory of Molecular Genetics and Immunology, The Rockefeller University, 1230 York Ave, New York, NY 10065, USA
e-mail: sbournazos@rockefeller.edu

Current Topics in Microbiology and Immunology (2019) 423: 1–12
https://doi.org/10.1007/82_2019_149
© Springer Nature Switzerland AG 2019
Published online: 10 February 2019

various leukocyte populations, as well as affinity for human IgGs. Such inter-species differences in FcγRs biology between humans and other mammalian species represents a major limitation for the interpretation of in vivo studies on human IgG function using conventional animal models.

1 The Emergence of IgG Antibodies

Complex defense mechanisms are ubiquitously found in all living organisms and are critical for the survival of these organisms in an antigenic world. Immunity is generally mediated by the early reactions of the innate immune system, followed by the later responses of adaptive immunity, characterized by almost infinite diversity and high specificity. Although immune mechanisms featuring the cardinal signs of adaptive immunity, i.e. diversity and specificity, have been discovered in invertebrates and jawless vertebrates, adaptive immunity based on highly diversified antigen-specific receptors is present only in jawed vertebrates. Indeed, key immune components of adaptive immunity, including antigen receptors, such as immunoglobulins (Ig) and T-cell receptors (TCR), as well as antigen-presenting MHC molecules are locked in a coevolving unit that orchestrates clonal selection and MHC-regulated processes during an adaptive immune response.

In addition to their common function, adaptive immune antigen receptors, such as Ig and TCR, share structural similarities, as they both comprise domains of the immunoglobulin superfamily (IgSF). IgSF domains are the building blocks for a large number of molecules across several species of the animal kingdom and represent the most prevalent domain in immune defense molecules. Apart from antigen receptors, IgSF domains are found in numerous receptors and molecules with a key role in cell-cell interactions, cell adhesion, as well as immune cell signaling. Despite the diverse functions of IgSF-containing molecules, these functions are somehow related, as IgSF domains are almost exclusively involved in protein-ligand interactions. The main structural feature of the IgSF domain is the stable shape of a β barrel that comprises two interfacing β sheets that are typically linked by a disulfide bond. Based on the domain constitution of their β strands and loops, IgSF domains are classified into four major types: the variable (V), the two constant domains (C1 and C2), as well as an intermediate type, which shares common features with both the C1 and C2 domains. Among the IgSF domains, the V domain type is the most structurally flexible and complex, featuring more strands, which correspond to the CDR2 region in Ig and TCRs. These unique structural features are critical for mediating highly specific antigenic recognition, accommodating the high degree of sequence diversity that characterizes antigen receptors, such as Ig and TCRs. The final structure of these antigen receptors is achieved through a linear combination of V and C-type IgSF domains. For example, a typical Ig molecule is a heterodimeric structure that comprises two polypeptides of the heavy chain and two of the light chain that are linked via several disulfide bonds forming a macromolecular complex. Each light chain comprises a single V and a C1 IgSF domain, whereas the Ig heavy chain is formed through the joining of the V-type domain with three-four C1 IgSF domains; the exact number of C domains is variable among the different Ig isotypes.

These unique structural features are highly conserved among all the different Ig isotypes found in diverse species of jawed vertebrates. Indeed, IgM, which is present in all jawed vertebrates, and is thought to represent the primordial Ig isotype, consists of a heavy chain peptide with one V and four C1 domains, which pairs with the light chain (one V and one C1 IgSF domain) through multiple inter-chain disulfide bridges. Monomeric IgM subunits form pentamers or hexamers in the majority of vertebrate species, apart from teleost fish, which form tetramers. Comparative analysis of the Ig isotypes in the jawed vertebrates suggests that a common precursor isotype that is related to IgM and can be traced at the inception of adaptive immunity, gave rise to the various Ig isotypes in jawed vertebrates at specific divergence points during evolution. These Ig isotypes have evolved under constant selection pressure from the challenging antigenic conditions encountered by the various vertebrate species. Indeed, the different Ig isotypes exhibit unique structural and functional characteristics, as well as distinct expression patterns among the various tissue compartments (intestinal, mucosal, serum etc.). For mammalian species, IgG and IgE represent two Ig isotypes that are exclusively found in mammals and mediate effector functions during an adaptive immune response. These isotypes are thought to have emerged from a common, structurally-related ancestor molecule, IgY, which is present in other vertebrate classes, including birds, reptiles, and amphibians, and represents the most abundant, secreted Ig isotype in these species.

2 Evolution of FcγR Genes in Mammalian Species

Since the IgG isotype is exclusively found in mammals, receptors for IgG antibodies only exist in mammalian species. These receptors, termed Fcγ receptors (FcγRs), interact with the constant region of the IgG heavy chain heterodimer and have co-evolved in mammalian species along with the emergence of the IgG isotype. For mammals, IgG represents the major Ig isotype in circulation and is abundantly expressed during an adaptive immune response. By directly interacting with IgG antibodies, FcγRs are critical for mediating downstream effector activities with tremendous impact on diverse innate and adaptive pathways. Indeed, despite being a major component of adaptive immunity, IgG antibodies link the innate and adaptive branches of immunity through specific interactions with the FcγRs expressed on the surface of effector leukocytes. Such interactions initiate diverse signaling processes with pleiotropic immunomodulatory functions, which have significant consequences for several aspects of innate and adaptive immunity. Such functions include the regulation of innate leukocyte activation, the uptake of foreign antigens via phagocytic mechanisms and their processing and presentation to MHC molecules, the regulation of antigen-presenting cell function, the stimulation of cytokine and chemokine synthesis, as well as the selection of high-affinity B-cells, and the regulation of plasma cell survival and consequently IgG production (Bournazos et al. 2017).

Given the diverse immunomodulatory consequences of FcγR engagement by the Fc domain of IgG antibodies, a number of FcγRs have emerged during mammalian evolution, each with distinct signaling activity and function, as well as unique expression profile among the various leukocyte cell types. On the basis of their intracellular signaling motifs and their capacity to induce stimulatory or inhibitory signaling cascades, FcγRs are broadly classified into activating or inhibitory (Nimmerjahn and Ravetch 2005). The major determinant that controls the affinity of an IgG molecule for the various FcγR types is the intrinsic flexibility of the Fc domain of IgG (Pincetic et al. 2014). Similar to the structural characteristics of all Ig isotypes, IgG molecules comprise two heavy and two light chains that are linked into a heterodimeric macromolecular complex through inter-chain disulfide bonds. Each light chain comprises one V-type IgSF domain and a C1-type domain, whereas each heavy chain consists of one V-type domain followed by three C1-type domains, corresponding to the CH1–CH3 domains of the IgG molecule. The characteristic Y structure of the IgG molecule arises from the presence of a hinge domain that separates the Fab domain (CH1 and light chains) from the Fc domain, which comprises the CH2 and CH3 domains. The FcγR binding sites are mapped at the Fc domain at two distinct positions; Type I FcγRs engage the Fc domain at the hinge-proximal region of the CH2 domain, whereas type II FcγRs at the CH2–3 interface (Pincetic et al. 2014). FcγR binding is accomplished through the characteristic horseshoe-like conformation of the Fc domain, which is formed by the tight association of the two CH3 domains at the C-terminal proximal region of the IgG molecule, while the two CH2 domains remain spatially separated. This characteristic tertiary structure of the Fc domain is achieved through the presence of an N-linked glycan conjugated at the amino acid backbone of the CH2 domain of the two heavy chains. The amino acid residue, where this glycan is conjugated is highly conserved in all IgG subclasses from all mammalian species, highlighting the importance of this glycan structure in the regulation of the Fc domain structure and consequently in Fc-FcγR interactions. This Fc-associated glycan resides within the hydrophobic cleft formed by the two CH2 domains and its composition regulates the conformational flexibility of the Fc domain and its capacity to interact with the various type I and type II FcγRs (Sondermann et al. 2013). Indeed, the presence of this glycan structure is critical for maintaining the Fc domain structure permissive for Fc-FcγR interactions, as loss of this glycan either through enzymatic removal or mutation of the amino acid residue where this structure is conjugated diminishes the affinity of the IgG Fc domain for all FcγR types (Albert et al. 2008; Lux et al. 2013).

Although the presence of the Fc-associated glycan structure is critical for maintaining the conformational structure of the Fc domain, the precise composition of the Fc glycan represents a key regulatory mechanism that controls the affinity of the Fc domain for the various FcγR classes. More specifically, the Fc-associated glycan structure consists of a core biantennary heptasaccharide moiety, which can be modified through the conjugation of additional saccharide units (fucose, galactose, N-acetylglucosamine, sialic acid), thereby yielding numerous variants with differential capacity to modulate Fc domain flexibility and consequently the affinity for the various FcγR types (Bournazos et al. 2017). Analysis of the Fc-associated glycan structure in circulating IgG antibodies has previously revealed substantial heterogeneity with specific Fc glycoforms becoming enriched upon infection and vaccination, in metabolic disease, during pregnancy, as well as during the remission/relapse phases of autoimmune disorders (Anthony et al. 2012; Nakagawa et al. 2007; Scherer et al. 2010; Theodoratou et al. 2016; Wang et al. 2015). Apart from the structure and composition of the Fc-associated glycan, differences in the primary amino acid sequence between the various IgG subclasses represent an additional level of regulation for Fc-FcγR interactions. Although protein homology between subclasses is typically over 95%, differences that exist at the hinge proximal region of the CH2 domain, where the interface for Fc-FcγR interactions is mapped, account for the differential binding profile of the IgG subclasses for the various FcγR types. Such differences are evident in the IgG subclasses from all mammalian species and along with the composition of the Fc-associated glycan, represent the main determinants for regulating Fc-FcγR interactions.

In all mammalian species, IgG molecules share highly conserved structural characteristics that determine the capacity of the Fc domain to interact with the various FcγRs and regulate its affinity. As FcγRs have co-evolved with IgG molecules during the emergence of the mammalian class, they feature a number of highly conserved properties that are fundamental for their ligand binding and signaling activities. For example, type I FcγRs can transduce either activating or inhibitory signals upon engagement by the IgG Fc domain, which is accomplished through specialized signaling motifs at their intracellular domains (Bournazos et al. 2017). Activating type I FcγRs feature intracellular tyrosine activating motifs (ITAMs) at their cytoplasmic domains, which transduce cell activating signals upon receptor crosslinking by the Fc domains of IgG immune complexes. Such signaling motifs are highly conserved among mammalian species and several innate and adaptive immunoreceptors, including TCRs, depend on ITAM-mediated signaling for their function. Activating type I FcγR-mediated signaling is counterbalanced by inhibitory FcγRs, whose cytoplasmic domains comprise intracellular tyrosine inhibition motifs (ITIMs) that associate with tyrosine phosphatases to inhibit kinase activity. The balancing activity of ITAM- and ITIM-containing FcγRs represents a key homeostatic mechanism that controls IgG-mediated inflammation and limits excessive or inappropriate cellular activation. Indeed, in nearly all effector leukocytes, activating type I FcγR expression is coupled with the expression of an inhibitory FcγR that regulates the signaling outcome of Fc-FcγR interactions. In addition to FcγRs, paired co-expression of activating and inhibitory immunoreceptors is very commonly found in several immune pathways, representing a fundamental mechanism for the control a number of processes of the innate and adaptive immunity.

In addition to the intracellular motifs and the downstream components that are required for the signal transduction of FcγRs, the FcγR ligand binding domains share highly homologous features among mammalian species. All type I FcγRs are members of the IgSF and their extracellular, IgG-binding domain consists of two (or three for the high-affinity FcγRI) C2-type IgSF domains. On the contrary, type II FcγRs are not structurally related to type I FcγRs, as their extracellular domain belongs to the C-type lectin family of receptors. Consistent with the structural differences in their extracellular, ligand-binding domains, type I and type II FcγRs engage the IgG Fc domain at distinct, non-overlapping regions; the hinge-proximal region of CH2 serves as the binding site for type I FcγRs, whereas type II FcγRs engage the Fc domain at the CH2–3 interface in a 2:1 (receptor:IgG) binding stoichiometry (Sondermann et al. 2013). In humans, several genes, each with multiple transcriptional isoforms, encode the different type I and type II FcγRs (Pincetic et al. 2014). Consistent with their common functional properties, members of the type I and type II FcγRs are mapped at specific loci on human chromosome 1 (1q23) and 19 (19p13), respectively. Clustering of the various human FcγR genes at specific genomic loci, along with the high degree of sequence homology between members of the same FcγR type, suggest that mammalian FcγR genes have emerged from a common ancestral precursor gene. Indeed, comparative analysis of the type I FcγR gene locus among different mammalian species shows a high degree of sequence homology, indicative of the emergence of this locus very early in mammalian evolutionary history (Fig. 1). This locus consists of three type I FcγR genes, corresponding to the human *FCGR2A*, *FCGR3A*, and *FCGR2B* genes. The genomic organization of this locus is conserved among diverse mammalian species, from very primitive mammals to primates, except for humans and chimpanzees. Due to the high sequence similarity of the ancestral *FCGR2A* and *FCGR2B* genes, sequential non-homologous recombination events that occurred late in human and chimpanzee divergence from the common non-human primate ancestor generated additional type I FcγR genes (Qiu et al. 1990) (Fig. 2). These genes are uniquely found in humans and chimpanzees and include *FCGR2C* and *FCGR3B*, which encode for FcγRIIc and FcγRIIIb, respectively. *FCGR3B* originates from a gene duplication event of *FCGR3A* and both genes share a very high degree of sequence homology. However, contrary to FcγRIIIa, FcγRIIIb is processed as a GPI-anchored molecule and lacks an intracellular domain; an effect attributed to the presence of a single nucleotide substitution (F203S) within the *FCGR3B* coding sequence. This point mutation is mapped at the membrane proximal region of the extracellular domain of FcγRIIIb and creates a post-translational modification signal sequence that processes FcγRIIIb as a GPI-anchored protein. Another type I FcγR gene that is uniquely found in humans and chimpanzees is *FCGR2C*, which is the result of the non-homologous recombination between the *FCGR2A* and *FCGR2B* genes. *FCGR2C* is essentially a

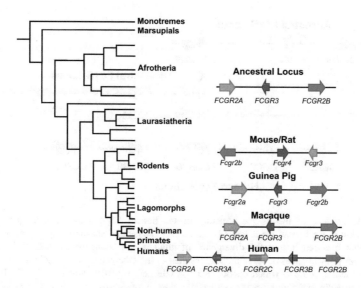

Fig. 1 Evolutionary conservation of the FcγR locus among mammalian species. The ancestral FcγR locus comprises three low-affinity FcγR genes that encode two activating (*FCGR2A* and *FCGR3*) and one inhibitory FcγRs (*FCGR2B*). These FcγRs feature two extracellular C2-type IgSF domains that mediate the recognition of the IgG Fc domain. This ancestral locus shares a common genomic structure and exhibits high sequence homology in diverse mammalian species, including non-human primates, like rhesus macaques. However, in humans and chimpanzees, the FcγR locus features unique characteristics and comprises additional FcγR genes (*FCGR2C* and *FCGR3B*)

chimeric gene, which comprises the exons that encode the extracellular domain of FcγRIIb, whereas the transmembrane and intracellular domains originate from FcγRIIa.

3 Inter-species Differences and Limitations for the Study of Human FcγR Function

Differences in the FcγR biology between humans and other mammalian species are not limited to the unique organization of the human FcγR locus and the presence of additional FcγR genes, like *FCGR3B* and *FCGR2C*, but extend to the FcγR structural characteristics and expression pattern among the various leukocyte cell types. For example, in murine species, all activating FcγRs require the FcR γ-chain for expression, assembly to the cell membrane, and signaling, whereas, in humans, FcγRIIa and FcγRIIc expression and signaling is not dependent on FcR γ-chain expression, as the cytoplasmic domains of these FcγRs contain ITAMs that can sufficiently transduce signals upon receptor engagement. FcγRIIIb, which is exclusively expressed in humans, has a unique structure that is not found in any

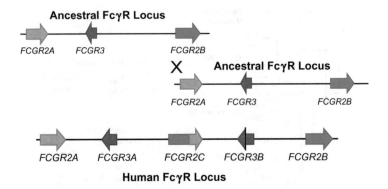

Fig. 2 Emergence of the unique structure of the human FcγR locus. The unique genomic organization of the human FcγR locus is attributed to sequential non-homologous recombination events that occurred late in the divergence of humans and chimpanzees from their common non-human primate ancestor. This process resulted in the emergence of two unique FcγR genes: *FCGR2C* and *FCGR3B*, which encode for FcγRIIc and FcγRIIIb, respectively. FcγRIIc is a chimeric receptor that comprises the extracellular domain of FcγRIIb, whereas the transmembrane and intracellular domains originate from FcγRIIa. FcγRIIIb shares high sequence homology with FcγRIIIa; however, FcγRIIIb is processed as a GPI-anchored molecule, lacking an intracellular domain

other FcγR, as it is processed as a GPI-anchored protein, lacking a transmembrane domain. As a consequence, FcγRIIIb cannot transduce any signals following crosslinking by IgG immune complexes; however, it is preferentially localized in lipid rafts microdomains that are enriched in membrane-associated kinases, and might utilize such signal transduction machinery to initiate intrinsic signals upon receptor engagement (Zhou and Brown 1994; Unkeless et al. 1995). Additionally, the FcγR expression pattern differs dramatically between humans and other mammalian species, including murine and non-human primates (Table 1). For example, human neutrophils express FcγRIIa, FcγRIIb, and FcγRIIIb, whereas neutrophils from non-human primates express FcγRI, FcγRIIa, and FcγRIIb. Likewise, at steady state conditions, monocyte-derived dendritic cells from humans express only FcγRIIa and FcγRIIb, whereas their murine counterparts express the full array of murine FcγRs, including FcγRI, FcγRIIb, FcγRIII, and FcγRIV.

These substantial inter-species differences in the FcγR genomic organization, structure, and function, as well as expression pattern, represent a major obstacle for the study of human IgG antibody function in vivo using conventional experimental animal model systems. Indeed, none of the commonly used experimental species, including mice, guinea pigs, rats, and non-human primates, can mirror precisely the structural diversity, IgG binding affinity, and the unique expression pattern for human FcγRs on human cells (Bournazos et al. 2015). Therefore, the use of such strains provides limited information on the role of human IgG Fc-FcγR interactions in the in vivo function of antibodies and cannot guide the development and pre-clinical evaluation of human IgG antibodies intended for clinical use in humans.

Table 1 FcγR expression pattern in effector leukocytes among humans, murine and non-human primate species

		FcγRI	FcγRIIa*	FcγRIIb	FcγRIIc#	FcγRIIIa**	FcγRIIIb#
NK cells	Human	-	-	-	++	+++	-
	Rhesus	-	-	-		+	
	Mouse	-	++	-		-	
Monocytes	Human	+++	++	+++	-	-/++	-
	Rhesus	++++	+	+		-/+	
	Mouse	+++	++	+++		++	
Neutrophils	Human	-	+++	+	-	-	+++++
	Rhesus	++++	++++	++		-	
	Mouse	++	++	+		+++	
B cells	Human	-	-	++++	-	-	-
	Rhesus	-	-	-/+		-	
	Mouse	-	-	++++		-	
* FcγRIII in murine species; ** FcγRIV in murine species; # human only							

Such limitation also applies to studies aiming to evaluate the in vivo activity of human-derived polyclonal IgG antibodies. More specifically, it is estimated that in human circulation, over 10^3 different Fc domain variants exist, stemming from differences in the amino acid sequence of the four IgG subclass and in the structure and composition of the Fc-associated glycan. These Fc variants display differential affinity for the various FcγR types, thereby exhibiting variable immunomodulatory activity (Bournazos et al. 2017). Such differences in the FcγR affinity among the human Fc domain variants present in circulation are specific for human FcγRs and do not extend to FcγRs from other species. Therefore, any studies aiming either to dissect the role of human-derived IgGs or to pre-clinically evaluate human IgG antibody therapeutics, necessitate the use of species-matched IgG-FcγR conditions.

To overcome this problem, during the past few years there have been efforts to generate mouse strains that express all human FcγRs in lieu of their mouse counterparts. Such FcγR humanized mouse model has been generated through the specific deletion of the genes that encode the mouse FcγRs and the introduction of all human FcγR genes as BAC transgenes under the control of their endogenous promoters and regulatory elements (Smith et al. 2012). Characterization of the FcγR expression levels and distribution among the various leukocyte populations revealed that FcγR humanized mice exhibited an FcγR expression pattern identical to that of humans (Smith et al. 2012). More importantly, these mice faithfully recapitulate the functional activity of human FcγRs in vivo and have been used in numerous studies to evaluate the in vivo activity of human therapeutic antibodies against infectious and neoplastic disorders (Bournazos et al. 2017; Li et al. 2017; Dahan et al. 2016; Georgoudaki et al. 2016; Lu et al. 2016; Dahan et al. 2015; DiLillo and Ravetch 2015; Bournazos et al. 2014a, b, DiLillo et al. 2014; Li et al. 2014; Li and Ravetch 2013).

4 Concluding Remarks

Along with the emergence of the IgG molecule, as the major Ig isotype elicited upon antigenic challenge, several FcγRs have evolved in mammalian species to interact with the Fc domain of IgG and mediate effector activity by directly linking IgGs to effector leukocytes. Even among diverse mammalian species, FcγRs are highly conserved and share a number of structural and functional features necessary for their ligand binding and signaling activities. Despite the high degree of sequence homology between FcγRs from different mammalian species, human FcγRs exhibit unique features related to the expression pattern among the various leukocyte cell types, as well as to the affinity for the different IgG Fc domain variants. These substantial inter-species differences represent major limitations for the accurate evaluation of human IgG function in vivo, as none of the conventional animal models can replicate the unique structural and functional diversity of human FcγRs. In-depth understanding of the evolutionary history of the FcγR-encoding genes, along with the thorough characterization of the unique features of FcγR of different mammalian species is essential for the design and interpretation of studies on IgG function in mammalian strains that are commonly used as disease models.

References

Albert H, Collin M, Dudziak D, Ravetch JV, Nimmerjahn F (2008) In vivo enzymatic modulation of IgG glycosylation inhibits autoimmune disease in an IgG subclass-dependent manner. Proc Natl Acad Sci U S A 105:15005–15009

Anthony RM, Wermeling F, Ravetch JV (2012) Novel roles for the IgG Fc glycan. Ann N Y Acad Sci 1253:170–180

Bournazos S, Chow SK, Abboud N, Casadevall A, Ravetch JV (2014a) Human IgG Fc domain engineering enhances antitoxin neutralizing antibody activity. J Clin Invest 124:725–729

Bournazos S, Klein F, Pietzsch J, Seaman MS, Nussenzweig MC, Ravetch JV (2014b) Broadly neutralizing anti-HIV-1 antibodies require Fc effector functions for in vivo activity. Cell 158:1243–1253

Bournazos S, DiLillo DJ, Ravetch JV (2015) The role of Fc-FcγR interactions in IgG-mediated microbial neutralization. J Exp Med 212:1361–1369

Bournazos S, Wang TT, Dahan R, Maamary J, Ravetch JV (2017) Signaling by antibodies: recent progress. Annu Rev Immunol 35:285–311

Dahan R, Sega E, Engelhardt J, Selby M, Korman AJ, Ravetch JV (2015) FcγRs modulate the anti-tumor activity of antibodies targeting the PD-1/PD-L1 axis. Cancer Cell 28:285–295

Dahan R, Barnhart BC, Li F, Yamniuk AP, Korman AJ, Ravetch JV (2016) Therapeutic activity of agonistic, human anti-CD40 monoclonal antibodies requires selective FcγR engagement. Cancer Cell 29:820–831

DiLillo DJ, Ravetch JV (2015) Differential Fc-receptor engagement drives an anti-tumor vaccinal effect. Cell 161:1035–1045

DiLillo DJ, Tan GS, Palese P, Ravetch JV (2014) Broadly neutralizing hemagglutinin stalk-specific antibodies require FcγR interactions for protection against influenza virus in vivo. Nat Med 20:143–151

Georgoudaki AM, Prokopec KE, Boura VF, Hellqvist E, Sohn S, Ostling J, Dahan R, Harris RA, Rantalainen M, Klevebring D, Sund M, Brage SE, Fuxe J, Rolny C, Li F, Ravetch JV, Karlsson MC (2016) Reprogramming tumor-associated macrophages by antibody targeting inhibits cancer progression and metastasis. Cell Rep 15:2000–2011

Li F, Ravetch JV (2013) Antitumor activities of agonistic anti-TNFR antibodies require differential FcγRIIB coengagement in vivo. Proc Natl Acad Sci U S A 110:19501–19506

Li F, Smith P, Ravetch JV (2014) Inhibitory Fcγ receptor is required for the maintenance of tolerance through distinct mechanisms. J Immunol 192:3021–3028

Li T, DiLillo DJ, Bournazos S, Giddens JP, Ravetch JV, Wang LX (2017) Modulating IgG effector function by Fc glycan engineering. Proc Natl Acad Sci U S A 114:3485–3490

Lu CL, Murakowski DK, Bournazos S, Schoofs T, Sarkar D, Halper-Stromberg A, Horwitz JA, Nogueira L, Golijanin J, Gazumyan A, Ravetch JV, Caskey M, Chakraborty AK, Nussenzweig MC (2016) Enhanced clearance of HIV-1-infected cells by broadly neutralizing antibodies against HIV-1 in vivo. Science 352:1001–1004

Lux A, Yu X, Scanlan CN, Nimmerjahn F (2013) Impact of immune complex size and glycosylation on IgG binding to human FcγRs. J Immunol 190:4315–4323

Nakagawa H, Hato M, Takegawa Y, Deguchi K, Ito H, Takahata M, Iwasaki N, Minami A, Nishimura S (2007) Detection of altered N-glycan profiles in whole serum from rheumatoid arthritis patients. J Chromatogr B Analyt Technol Biomed Life Sci 853:133–137

Nimmerjahn F, Ravetch JV (2005) Divergent immunoglobulin g subclass activity through selective Fc receptor binding. Science 310:1510–1512

Pincetic A, Bournazos S, DiLillo DJ, Maamary J, Wang TT, Dahan R, Fiebiger BM, Ravetch JV (2014) Type I and type II Fc receptors regulate innate and adaptive immunity. Nat Immunol 15:707–716

Qiu WQ, de Bruin D, Brownstein BH, Pearse R, Ravetch JV (1990) Organization of the human and mouse low-affinity Fc gamma R genes: duplication and recombination. Science 248: 732–735

Scherer HU, van der Woude D, Ioan-Facsinay A, el Bannoudi H, Trouw LA, Wang J, Häupl T, Burmester GR, Deelder AM, Huizinga TW, Wuhrer M, Toes RE (2010) Glycan profiling of anti-citrullinated protein antibodies isolated from human serum and synovial fluid. Arthritis Rheum 62:1620–1629

Smith P, DiLillo DJ, Bournazos S, Li F, Ravetch JV (2012) Mouse model recapitulating human Fcγ receptor structural and functional diversity. Proc Natl Acad Sci U S A 109:6181–6186

Sondermann P, Pincetic A, Maamary J, Lammens K, Ravetch JV (2013) General mechanism for modulating immunoglobulin effector function. Proc Natl Acad Sci U S A 110:9868–9872

Theodoratou E, Thaçi K, Agakov F, Timofeeva MN, Štambuk J, Pučić-Baković M, Vučković F, Orchard P, Agakova A, Din FV, Brown E, Rudd PM, Farrington SM, Dunlop MG, Campbell H, Lauc G (2016) Glycosylation of plasma IgG in colorectal cancer prognosis. Sci Rep 6:28098

Unkeless JC, Shen Z, Lin CW, DeBeus E (1995) Function of human Fc γ RIIA and Fc γ RIIIB. Semin Immunol 7:37–44

Wang TT, Maamary J, Tan GS, Bournazos S, Davis CW, Krammer F, Schlesinger SJ, Palese P, Ahmed R, Ravetch JV (2015) Anti-HA glycoforms drive B cell affinity selection and determine influenza vaccine efficacy. Cell 162:160–169

Zhou MJ, Brown EJ (1994) CR3 (Mac-1, alpha M beta 2, CD11b/CD18) and Fc gamma RIII cooperate in generation of a neutrophil respiratory burst: requirement for Fc gamma RIII and tyrosine phosphorylation. J Cell Biol 125:1407–1416

Role of FcγRs in Antibody-Based Cancer Therapy

Robert F. Graziano and John J. Engelhardt

Contents

Abstract Monoclonal antibodies can mediate antitumor activity by multiple mechanisms. They can bind directly to tumor receptors resulting in tumor cell death, or can bind to soluble growth factors, angiogenic factors, or their cognate receptors blocking signals required for tumor cell growth or survival. Monoclonal antibodies, upon binding to tumor cell, can also engage the host's immune system to mediate immune-mediated destruction of the tumor. The Fc portion of the antibody is essential in engaging the host immune system by fixing complement resulting in complement-mediated cytotoxicity (CDC) of the tumor, or by engaging Fc receptors for IgG (FcγR) expressed by leukocytes leading to antibody-dependent cellular cytotoxicity (ADCC) or antibody-dependent cellular phagocytosis (ADCP) of tumor cells. Antibodies whose Fc portion preferentially engage activating FcγRs have shown greater inhibition of tumor growth and metastasis. Monoclonal antibodies can also stimulate the immune system by binding to targets expressed on immune cells. These antibodies may stimulate antitumor immunity by antagonizing a negative regulatory signal, agonizing a costimulatory signal, or depleting immune

R. F. Graziano · J. J. Engelhardt (✉)
Oncology Discovery, Bristol-Myers Squibb, Princeton, NJ, Redwood City, CA, USA
e-mail: john.engelhardt@bms.com

Current Topics in Microbiology and Immunology (2019) 423: 13–34
https://doi.org/10.1007/82_2019_150
© Springer Nature Switzerland AG 2019
Published online: 22 February 2019

cells that are inhibitory. The importance of Fc:FcγR interactions in antitumor therapy for each of these mechanisms have been demonstrated in both mouse models and clinical trials and will be the focus of this chapter.

1 Introduction

The development of hybridoma technology described by Kohler and Milstein over 40 years ago triggered the concept of using monoclonal antibodies (mAbs) as therapeutic drugs (Köhler and Milstein 1975). However, largely due to immunogenicity and the short serum half-life of mouse antibodies in human patients, this potential was not immediately realized. Advances in molecular biology, antibody engineering, and transgenic mouse technology led to the development of chimeric (Boulianne et al. 1984; Morrison et al. 1984), humanized (Jones et al. 1986), and fully human(Taylor et al. 1992; Jakobovits 1998; Tuaillon et al. 1993) mAbs, which significantly reduced problems encountered with mouse mAbs. Rituximab, an anti-CD20 monoclonal antibody developed for the treatment of B cell non-Hodgkin's lymphoma (B-NHL) and chronic lymphocytic leukemia (CLL), was the first FDA-approved monoclonal antibody for cancer therapy (Maloney et al. 1997). Rituximab was FDA-approved in 1997 and since then more than 25 additional mAbs have been approved for treating cancer and many more are in clinical development. With further technological advancements in antibody engineering, tumor cell biology and cellular immunology came more innovative approaches to inhibiting cancer growth with one or more mAbs (reviewed further in (Weiner et al. 2009)).

Monoclonal antibodies can mediate their antitumor activity by several different, but not mutually exclusive, mechanisms. Monoclonal antibodies to VEGF or to VEGFR2 block the supply of blood to tumors by inhibiting angiogenesis (Ferrara et al. 2004; Lu et al. 2003). One class of mAbs that binds directly to tumor-associated antigens (TAA) can inhibit tumor growth by blocking a growth signal or by directly inducing tumor cell death. In addition, as the antigen-binding fragment (Fab) of the mAb binds to the TAA, the Fc portion of the mAb may engage the host immune system by fixing complement, resulting in complement-dependent cytotoxicity (CDC) of the tumor. The mAb can also bind to Fc receptors for IgG (FcγR) expressed on immune effector cells, which can result in antibody-dependent cellular cytotoxicity (ADCC) or antibody-dependent cellular phagocytosis (ADCP) of the tumor cell. ADCP mediated by dendritic cells or macrophages may also result in augmented antigen presentation to tumor-specific T cells, engaging cells of the adaptive immune system to eliminate tumors (DiLillo and Ravetch 2015).

Another class of therapeutic mAb binds to immune cells rather than the tumor cell, leading to enhanced immune activation. This type of antibody can mediate its effect by antagonizing a negative regulatory signal or by agonizing a costimulatory signal leading to prolonged and/or enhanced antitumor immunity. Recent evidence also suggests that mAb that bind to and deplete regulatory T cells (Treg) via ADCC or ADCP can also augment antitumor activity (Selby et al. 2013; Simpson et al.

2013). This review will focus on the importance of Fc:FcγR interactions in anti-tumor immunity.

1.1 Mouse FcγRs

Four FcγRs have been molecularly characterized in the mouse system: FcγRI, FcγRIIb, FcγRIII, and FcγRIV (Table 1). FcγRI, FcγRIII, and FcγRIV are activating receptors that are non-covalently associated with the immunoreceptor tyrosine-based activation motif (ITAM)-containing common γ-signaling chain. The activating receptors mediate ADCC and ADCP of antibody-opsonized target cells. Conversely, FcγRIIb is an inhibitory FcγR and contains an immunoreceptor tyrosine-based inhibitory motif (ITIM) in its intracellular domain. Engagement of this receptor can inhibit ADCC and ADCP. These four receptors have overlapping expression patterns as well as differing affinities for the Fc portion of the four mouse subclasses of IgG: IgG1, IgG2a, IgG2b, and IgG3. The Fc portion of antibodies of the IgG2a subclass, and to a lesser extent the IgG2b subclass, bind preferentially to the activating receptors FcγRI and FcγRIV, whereas antibodies of the IgG1 subclass have low affinity for these receptors. However, IgG1 mAb has higher affinity than IgG2a for the inhibitory FcγRIIb. IgG1, IgG2a, and IgG2b bind FcγRIII with similar affinities. The avidity of IgG3 for each of the FcγR is very low to non-detectable. As described in the following section, the preferential binding of tumor-specific IgG2a subclass mAb to activating FcγR results in increased antitumor efficacy in vivo (Nimmerjahn and Ravetch 2005; Ravetch and Lanier 2000), reviewed in (Clynes 2006)).

1.2 Human FcγRs

The human FcγR family has similarities to the mouse family but also differs in several significant ways. The human FcγR family does not contain a true homolog to the mouse FcγRIV and the mouse FcγR family does not contain a true homolog of the human FcγRIIa. FcγRIIa is an activating receptor that does not associate with the ITAM-containing common γ signaling chain, but contains an ITAM domain in its intracellular domain. In addition, two versions of human FcγRIII exist: FcγRIIIa, which contains a transmembrane region and associates with the ITAM-containing common γ signaling chain, and FcγRIIIb, which is a glycophosphatidylinositol (GPI)-linked FcγR and does not directly mediate an activating or inhibitory signal when engaged. Allelic variants of FcγRIIa and FcγRIIIa exist that have differing avidities for Fc. The H131 allelic version of FcγRIIa has overall higher affinity for Fc than the R131 allelic version and is the only FcγR with measurable affinity for the IgG2 subclass. The V158 allelic version of FcγRIIIa has overall higher avidity for Fc than the F158 allelic version (Bruhns et al. 2009; reviewed in Bruhns 2012) (Table 2).

Table 1 Mouse Fc receptors

FcγR	Affinity for huIgG	Isotype preference	Cellular distribution	Activating or inhibitory
FcγRI	High for IgG2a ($K_D \sim 10$ nM)	IgG2a $\ggg$ 2b $\gg$ 1, 3	Monocytes, macrophages, DCs	Activating, associates with ITAM-containing signaling chain
FcγRIIb	Low	IgG1 > 2b > 2a	B cells, neutrophils, monocytes, macrophages	Inhibitory, contains ITIM domain in ICD
FcγRIII	Low	IgG1 = 2a = 2b	NK cells, neutrophils, monocytes, macrophages, DCs	Activating, associates with ITAM-containing signaling chain
FcγRIV	Medium	IgG2a >= 2b	Neutrophils, monocytes, macrophages, DCs	Activating, associates with ITAM-containing signaling chain

Source Nimmerjahn and Ravetch, Science 2005

Unlike the varying selectivity of mouse IgG1 subclasses for binding to activating or inhibitory FcγRs, IgG1 in the human system IgG1 is the isotype that binds best to all types of FcγRs. Fc variants have been engineered by altering Fc glycosylation or by making amino acid substitutions that increase binding for specific FcγRs. Antibodies contain an N-linked glycosylation site at position 297. Antibodies engineered to lack fucose moieties in their glycan chain have higher affinity for both allelic versions of FcγRIIIA and mediate more potent ADCC and ADCP (Shields et al. 2002). Several amino acid-engineered variants of human IgG1 result in preferential enhanced affinity for activating FcγR and/or inhibitory FcγR, each of which may be utilized to enhance the activity of antitumor mAb, depending on the mechanism of action of the mAb (reviewed in (Barnhart and Quigley 2017)). These variants will be discussed throughout this review. Other alterations have been created to eliminate binding to complement and/or FcγR, resulting in an "inert" Fc (Tam et al. 2017; Clynes et al. 2000). A mAb with an inert Fc may be utilized when engagement of Fc effector mechanisms is undesirable, for example, to antagonize negative regulatory signals on effector T cells without depleting them.

2   Tumor-Targeting Antibodies

The importance of Fc:FcγR interactions in direct tumor targeting was established in early preclinical studies. Clynes et al. demonstrated that full in vivo activity of rituximab and trastuzumab required activating Fc:FcγR engagement (Clynes et al. 2000). Mice that were deficient in the γ signaling chain were unable to inhibit tumor growth in vivo compared to wild-type mice. Furthermore, engineered Fc versions of

Table 2 Human Fc Receptors

FcγR	Allelic variants	Affinity for huIgG	Isotype preference	Cellular distribution	Activating or inhibitory
FcγRI	None described	High ($K_D \sim 10$ nM)	IgG1 = 3 > 4 ≫ 2	Monocytes, macrophages, activated neutrophils, DCs	Activating, associates with ITAM-containing signaling chain
FcγRIIa	H131	Low to medium	IgG1 > 2 = 3 > 4	Neutrophils, monocytes, macrophages, eosinophils, DCs, platelets	Activating, contains ITAM domain in ICD
	R131	Low	IgG1 > 3 > 4 > 2		
FcγRIIb	I232	Low	IgG1 = 3 = 4 > 2	B cells, monocytes, macrophages, DCs, mast cells	Inhibitory, contains ITIM domain in ICD
	T232	Low	IgG1 = 3 = 4 > 2		
FcγRIIIa	V158	Medium	IgG1 = 3 ≫ 4 > 2	NK cells, monocytes, macrophages,, mast cells, eosinophils, DCs	Activating, associates with ITAM-containing signaling chain
	F158	Low	IgG1 = 3 ≫ 4 > 2		
FcγRIIIb	NA1	Low to medium	IgG1 = 3 ≫ 4 = 2	Neutrophils	Neutral, GPI-linked
	NA2	Low to medium	IgG1 = 3 ≫ 4 = 2		

these antibodies that were unable to engage FcγRs were also less active in eliminating tumors. These data implied that, of the various antitumor activities attributed to these mAbs (Table 3), FcγR-mediated ADCC/ADCP was the most relevant for efficacy in mouse tumor models and perhaps in treated patients. The authors also demonstrated that mice deficient in the inhibitory FcγR, FcγRIIB, were more capable of eliminating melanoma metastases than wild-type animals when treated with a mAb to the melanoma TAA, gp75. This finding suggested that the optimal design of antitumor mAb would preferentially engage activating FcγR and not inhibitory FcγR. It was subsequently shown that TAA-specific mAbs, with mouse Fcs that preferentially bind activating FcγRs relative to inhibitory FcγRs, were significantly more potent in their ability to inhibit tumor growth and metastasis in vivo. This suggested that isotypes that engage FcγR with a high activating to inhibitory ratio (A/I) accounted for this difference in activity (Ravetch and Lanier 2000; Nimmerjahn and Ravetch 2005).

Results from clinical studies also point to the importance of ADCC/ADCP in the efficacy of antitumor mAb. In patients with lymphoma, expression of high-affinity alleles of FcγRIIIa (FcγRIIIa-158 V) and FcγRIIa (FcγRIIa-131H) is associated with improved response to rituximab therapy, likely due to enhanced ADCC and/or ADCP (Cartron et al. 2002; Weng and Levy 2003). In fact, second-generation

Table 3 FDA-approved monoclonal antibodies for cancer therapy 1997–2018

Generic name	Trade name	Target	Fc format	Cancer	Target class	Purported MoA(s)	References
Rituximab	Rituxan	CD20	Chimeric mouse/human IgG1	B-NHL, CLL	Tumor	Direct tumor growth inhibition, CDC, ADCC, ADCP	Reviewed in Pierpont et al. (2018)
Ofatamumab	Arzerra	CD20	Human IgG1	CLL	Tumor	Direct tumor growth inhibition, CDC, ADCC, ADCP	Osterborg et al. (2016)
Obinutuzumab	Gazyva	CD20	Humanized IgG1 (nonfucosylated Fc)	B-NHL, CLL	Tumor	Direct tumor growth inhibition, CDC, eADCC, eADCP	Goede et al. (2014) and Salles et al. (2012)
Ibritumomab	Zevalin	CD20	Mouse IgG1 ^{90}Y-labeled	B-NHL	Tumor	Delivery of a toxic radioisotope to tumor	Grillo-Lopez (2002)
Alemtuzumab	Campath*	CD52	Humanized IgG1	B-CLL[a]	Tumor	Direct tumor growth inhibition, CDC, ADCC, ADCP?	Lundin et al. (1998)
Brentuximab vedotin	Adcetris	CD30	Chimeric mouse/human IgG1	HL, ALCL	Tumor	Delivery of a toxic payload to tumor	(Younes et al. 2010)
Gemtuzumab ozogamicin	Myelotarg	CD33	Humanized IgG4 ADC	AML	Tumor	Delivery of a toxic payload to tumor	Reviewed in Gbadamosi et al. (2018)
Inotuzumab ozogamicin	Besponsa	CD22	Humanized IgG4 ADC	ALL	Tumor	Delivery of a toxic payload to tumor	Reviewed in Tvito and Rowe (2017)
Trastuzumab	Herceptin	HER2	Humanized IgG1	Breast, stomach	Tumor	Direct tumor growth inhibition, ADCC, ADCP	Albanell and Baselga (1999)

(continued)

Table 3 (continued)

Generic name	Trade name	Target	Fc format	Cancer	Target class	Purported MoA(s)	References
Trastuzumab-dkst	Ogivri	HER2	Humanized IgG1	Breast, stomach	Tumor	Direct tumor growth inhibition, ADCC, ADCP	Serna-Gallegos et al. (2018)
ado-Trastuzumab-emtansine	Kadcyla	HER2	Humanized IgG1 ADC	Breast	Tumor	Delivery of a toxic payload to tumor	Amiri-Kordestani et al. (2014a)
Pertuzumab	Perjeta	HER2	Humanized IgG1	Breast	Tumor	Direct tumor growth inhibition, ADCC, ADCP	Amiri-Kordestani et al. (2014b)
Cetuximab	Erbitux	EGFR	Chimeric mouse/human IgG1	CRC, H&N	Tumor	Direct tumor growth inhibition, ADCC, ADCP	Reviewed in Goldberg (2005)
Panitumumab	Vectibix	EGFR	Human IgG2	CRC	Tumor	Direct tumor growth inhibition, ADCC, ADCP	Giusti et al. (2007)
Necitumumab	Portrazza	EGFR	Human IgG1	Lung	Tumor	Direct tumor growth inhibition, ADCC, ADCP	Dienstmann and Tabernero (2010)
Dinutuximab	Unituxin	GD2	Chimeric mouse/human IgG1	Neuroblastoma	Tumor	ADCC, ADCP	Dhillon (2015)
Olaratumab	Lartruvo	PDGFRA	Human IgG1	Sarcoma	Tumor	Direct tumor growth inhibition, ADCC, ADCP	Shirley (2017)
Bevacizumab	Avastin	VEGF	Humanized IgG1	CRC, lung, brain, kidney, cervical, ovarian	Growth factor	Inhibition of angiogenesis	Kerr (2004)

(continued)

Table 3 (continued)

Generic name	Trade name	Target	Fc format	Cancer	Target class	Purported MoA(s)	References
Bevacizumab-awwb	Mvasi	VEGF	Humanized IgG1	CRC, lung, brain, kidney, cervical	Growth factor	Inhibition of angiogenesis	Serna-Gallegos et al. (2018)
Ramucirumab	Cyramza	VEGFR2	Human IgG1	Stomach, CRC	Growth factor receptor, endothelial cell	Inhibition of angiogenesis	Poole and Vaidya (2014)
Elotuzumab	Empliciti	SLAMF7	Humanized IgG1	Multiple myeloma	Tumor, immune cell	ADCC, ADCP, activation of NK cells	Markham (2016)
Daratumumab	Darzalex	CD38	Human IgG1	Multiple myeloma	Tumor, immune cell	Direct tumor growth inhibition, ADCC, ADCP, depletion of Tregs	McKeage (2016)
Ipilimumab	Yervoy	CTLA-4	Human IgG1	Melanoma	Immune cell	Checkpoint blockade, depletion of Tregs	Cameron et al. (2011)
Nivolumab	Opdivo	PD-1	Human IgG4	Melanoma, CRC, kidney, lung, H&N, bladder, liver, HL	Immune cell	Checkpoint blockade	Kazandjian et al. (2016)
Pembrolizumab	Keytruda	PD-1	Humanized IgG4	Melanoma, CRC, stomach, lung, H&N, bladder, liver, HL	Immune cell	Checkpoint blockade	Poole (2014)
Atezolizumab	Tecentriq	PD-L1	Human IgG1 (engineered "inert" Fc)	Bladder, lung	Tumor, immune cell	Checkpoint blockade	Blair (2018)

(continued)

Table 3 (continued)

Generic name	Trade name	Target	Fc format	Cancer	Target class	Purported MoA(s)	References
Avelumab	Bavencio	PD-L1	Human IgG1	Merkel cell carcinoma	Tumor, immune cell	Checkpoint blockade	Kim (2017)
Durvalumab	Imfinzi	PD-L1	Human IgG1 (engineered "inert" Fc)	Bladder	Tumor, immune cell	Checkpoint blockade	Syed (2017)
Mogamulizumab-kpkc	Poteligeo	CCR4	IgG1-NF	CTCL	Tumor	Direct tumor growth inhibition, ADCC?	Kim et al. (2018)

[a]Campath was withdrawn from market as an agent for treating B-CLL in 2012 and subsequently approved for multiple sclerosis in 2014

anti-CD20 mAbs have been created that increase affinity for activating FcγR (Table 3). Ocaratuzumab is an IgG1 anti-human CD20 antibody in which two amino-acid substitutions were made in the human IgG1 Fc in order to increase affinity to both 158 V and 158F allotypes of FcγRIIIA (Forero-Torres et al. 2012; Klein et al. 2013). The enhanced FcγRIIIA binding and increased affinity to human CD20 have resulted in increased in vitro ADCC activity regardless of donor FcγRIIIA allotype. In addition, promising clinical responses have been seen in patients with follicular lymphoma, including patients who received prior rituximab and those harboring the 158F allotype of FcγRIIIA (Forero-Torres et al. 2012; Cheney et al. 2014; Tobinai et al. 2011).

Nonfucosylated antibodies can be generated via mutations at N-linked glycosylation sites in the Fc or a cell line lacking fucosyltransferases and fucose transporters (Yamane-Ohnuki and Satoh 2009). Increased function can be achieved with a nonfucosylated antibody, as demonstrated by clinical responses to rituximab (anti-human CD20 with wild-type IgG1) and obinutuzumab (anti-human CD20 with a nonfucosylated IgG1). Compared with rituximab plus chemotherapy, nonfucosylated obinutuzumab plus chemotherapy has demonstrated greater response rate and survival in patients with chronic lymphocytic leukemia (Goede et al. 2014). As observed with rituximab, patients who are homozygous for the 158 V allotype of FcγRIIIA tend to have stronger responses to obinutuzumab (Salles et al. 2012).

Recently two monoclonal antibodies received FDA approval for the treatment of multiple myeloma (MM). Daratumumab is a human IgG1 antibody that binds to CD38, which is expressed at high levels on the surface of MM tumors. Daratumumab manifests its activity through multiple mechanisms including CDC, ADCC, and ADCP of MM tumor cells (van der Veer et al. 2011; Overdijk et al. 2015). In addition to being expressed on MM tumor cells, CD38 is expressed on normal T cells, monocytes, B cells, NK cells, and, importantly, at high levels on Tregs, Bregs, and myeloid-derived suppressor cells (MDSC). An additional mechanism of action of daratumumab is to deplete Treg, Breg, and MDSC, cells that inhibit the antitumor immunity (Krejcik et al. 2016). This mechanism of action will be discussed in detail later in this review. A second monoclonal antibody that received FDA approval for the treatment of MM is elotuzumab (Lonial et al. 2015). Elotuzumab is a humanized IgG1 antibody that binds to SLAMF7, another receptor that is expressed at high levels on MM tumor cells. Elotuzumab was shown to mediate ADCC and ADCP of SLAMF7-expressing MM tumor cell lines in vitro (Hsi et al. 2008; Tai et al. 2008). SLAMF7 is also expressed as an activating receptor on normal NK cells, and binding of elotuzumab to NK cells can activate these effector cells to control tumor growth (Bouchon et al. 2001; Collins et al. 2013). Elotuzumab treatment inhibits tumor growth of human SLAMF7 positive MM tumor xenografts in immunocompromised mice (Hsi et al. 2008; Tai et al. 2008). This efficacy is dependent on FcγRIII engagement on NK cells—depletion of NK cells or blocking FcγRIII abrogates its efficacy (Hsi et al. 2008). In clinical studies, similar to what was observed with rituximab, benefits in progression-free survival were reported in patients with relapsed/refractory multiple myeloma (RRMM) who were homozygous for the FcγRIIIa-158 V allele and treated with elotuzumab in combination with bortezomib and dexamethasone (Jakubowiak et al. 2016).

FcγRs are expressed on cells of the innate immune system and, as discussed above, innate effector cells such as NK cells and myeloid cells are often required for the therapeutic efficacy of tumor-targeted mAbs in mouse tumor models. However, some studies of immunocompetent mice with syngeneic tumor allografts showed that depletion of cells of the adaptive immune response, in particular $CD8^+$ T cells, reduced the therapeutic effects of tumor-targeted mAbs (Kohrt et al. 2012; Park et al. 2010; Stagg et al. 2011). Furthermore, patients with lymphoma have developed lymphoma-specific $CD4^+$ and $CD8^+$ T cell responses after rituximab treatment, suggesting that tumor-targeted mAbs may initiate an antitumor adaptive immune response (Abès et al. 2010 #244). Experiments combining mAb to TAA with agents that antagonize immune checkpoints or agonize costimulatory receptors on the surface of T cells have been performed in mouse tumor models. For example, Stagg et al. (2011) demonstrated that the efficacy of an anti-HER2 antibody was dependent on NK cells and $CD8^+$ T cells and on release of type I and type II interferons. Furthermore, the combination of the anti-HER2 antibody with anti-PD-1 or anti-CD137 mAb enhanced antitumor efficacy toward HER2 + tumors versus single agents. Bezman et al. (Bezman et al. 2017) used mouse tumor cell lines that were engineered to express human SLAMF7 to look at the ability of the mouse IgG2a version of elotuzumab (elotuzumab-g2a) to reduce or eliminate tumor growth in immunocompetent mouse models. They showed that antitumor efficacy required both FcγRIII-expressing NK cells and $CD8^+$ T cells and was significantly enhanced by co-administration of anti-PD-1 antibody. Elotuzumab-g2a and anti-PD-1 combination treatment promoted tumor-infiltrating NK and $CD8^+$ T cell activation, as well as increased intratumoral cytokine and chemokine release.

3 Antibodies Against Immune Targets

In addition to directly targeting antigens expressed by tumor cells, antibodies are also used to influence the function of cells of the immune system. Antibodies against immune targets can be separated into three main mechanisms: antagonists, agonists, or depleting mAbs. In some cases, it is unclear whether more than one of these strategies is associated with a particular mAb, and Fc:FcγR interactions or lack thereof can determine which effect is occurring.

3.1 Depleting Antibodies: Regulatory T-Cell Targets

Anti-CTLA-4 treatment was the first example of an immune cell-targeted mAb having antitumor efficacy in mouse models (Leach et al. 1996). This finding was later translated to clinical treatment of patients with ipilimumab, the first checkpoint inhibitor approved for the treatment of human cancer. While the success of treatment with anti-CTLA-4 was originally attributed to blockade of CTLA-4 binding to its ligands CD80 and CD86, recent data have called that conclusion into question. Studies by three different research groups implicated the depletion of tumor-infiltrating Treg cells as being critical for the activity of anti-CTLA-4 in mouse tumor models. In Selby et al., the anti-mouse CTLA-4 mAb 9D9 (mouse IgG2b) was reformatted as multiple different isotypes (mIgG1 D265A, mIgG1, mIgG2a) to determine the role of Fc:FcR interactions on antitumor efficacy (Selby et al. 2013). Antitumor effects were found to correlate with the ability to engage activating FcγRs, i.e., the mIgG2a, which bound best to activating receptors, had the highest activity, and was followed by the original mIgG2b. The mIgG1 D265A isotype, which does not bind FcγRs, had no antitumor activity, and neither did the mIgG1, which preferentially binds to the inhibitory FcγRIIb. When the tumors of treated mice were examined by flow cytometry, it was found that Tregs were specifically reduced by the IgG2a isotype and to a lesser extent by the IgG2b isotype but not the mIgG1 or mIgG1 D265A. Depletion of peripheral Tregs in the spleen, lymph node or blood was not observed for any of the mAbs. Taken together this data revealed that binding to activating FcγRs was critical to the activity of anti-CTLA-4 treatment, and that blockade in the absence of Treg depletion had little to no antitumor activity.

In complementary work, Simpson et al. examined the effects of another anti-CTLA-4 mAb, 9H10, which is a hamster anti-mouse CTLA-4 mAb. Using an antigen-specific T-cell transfer system, they were able to demonstrate that 9H10 depleted tumor antigen-specific Tregs and also reduced endogenous Tregs (Simpson et al. 2013). Depletion was not changed when the experiments were performed in C3 KO mice or when NK cells were depleted, suggesting that complement or NK cells were not responsible for depletion. However, depletion was reduced in either Fcγ or FcγRIV KO mice, but not in FcγRIII KO mice. FcγRIV-expressing phagocytes were found to be more prevalent in the tumor microenvironment and, taken together with the lack of a role for NK cells in the process, FcγRIV-expressing macrophages/monocytes are implicated as the responsible effector cell population. Considering the results from these two papers, two different anti-mouse CTLA-4 mAbs, 9D9 and 9H10, were shown to deplete Tregs, and this effect was shown in three different mouse tumor models—MC38, CT26, and B16. The strength of this finding across different mAbs and models suggests this is indeed a critical mediator of antitumor efficacy in mice.

In another recent publication, Bulliard et al. also showed that efficacy and Treg depletion depended on isotype for both anti-CTLA-4 and anti-GITR mAbs (Bulliard et al. 2013). The finding that depletion of immune suppressive cells is also the primary mechanism of action of another T cell-directed antibody therapy confirms that this is a potent effector mechanism. Because GITR is a costimulatory receptor, antitumor efficacy mediated by the GITR mAb, DTA-1, was originally attributed to agonist activity against the receptor (Ko et al. 2005), but depletion of Tregs was later identified by Coe et al. (Coe et al. 2010). Determining that efficacy is dependent on ADCC of Tregs challenges this assumption and suggests that activity of antibodies against other T-cell costimulatory receptors should be re-evaluated.

Indeed, it has been found that mAbs against other receptors such as OX-40 (Bulliard et al. 2014), and ICOS are most efficacious when they mediate Treg depletion. While it is clear that mAbs against multiple T-cell surface receptors can mediate depletion of Tregs, it is less clear what effects these mAbs have on effector T-cell populations that can also express the receptors. Bulliard et al. noted reduction of effector CD4 s and CD8 s after both GITR and CTLA-4 mAb treatments, but this effect was not observed by Selby and Simpson for CTLA-4 or by Mahne for GITR (Mahne et al. 2017). However, the fact that no difference in abundance of bulk effector T cells was observed does not necessarily rule out an effect on effectors. Some effectors may be depleted by antibody treatment, but since Treg depletion would likely be inducing effector expansion separately, that expansion may mask some amount of effector depletion. Both GITR and CTLA-4 are expressed at higher levels on Treg cells than effector T cells, so this difference may result in preferential depletion of Tregs.

In addition to the costimulatory receptors described above, chemokine receptors are also being investigated as targets that can induce depletion of Treg cells. Two in particular have drawn increased attention. The chemokine receptor CCR4 is currently being targeted by the nonfucosylated mAb mogamulizumab. This mAb was originally developed for the treatment of cutaneous T-cell lymphoma, which expresses CCR4, but was also found to deplete Tregs from peripheral blood of patients treated with the mAb (Ogura et al. 2014). This has prompted testing of the mAb for treatment of solid tumors in addition to its original indication. However, CCR4 expression is not only found on Treg cells but also effector CD4 T cells, which could limit clinical activity due to depletion of these effectors in addition to Tregs. Plitas et al. recently identified another chemokine receptor, CCR8 that is more highly expressed by Treg cells at the tumor site compared to those in peripheral blood or tissues (Plitas et al. 2016). The CCR8 + Tregs appear to be the most activated Tregs, and CD4 and CD8 effector cells express little to no CCR8. These attributes make CCR8 an intriguing target that may avoid significant depletion of either peripheral Tregs or activated effector cells from the tumor site.

While the discovery of Treg depletion in mouse models suggests that this is a powerful means to improve immune responses to tumors, it also brings up important questions about how this process may occur in patients. Mouse syngeneic models are useful for determining antitumor efficacy of mAb therapies and were critical in demonstrating how both anti-CTLA-4 and anti-PD-1/L1 could enhance immune responses to tumors. However, extrapolating from the interactions of mouse Fc regions with mouse FcγRs to those of human Fcs and human FcγRs is not straightforward.

A critical tool for studying human Fc-FcR interactions in the context of mouse tumor model is the human FcR transgenic mouse model developed by Ravetch et al. These mice have had the mouse FcγRs knocked out, and the human FcγRs introduced transgenically (Smith et al. 2012). The mice thus express only human FcγRs and can be used to model the effect of human Fcs on the function of therapeutic mAbs. These mice have been used to investigate the roles of human Fcs on therapeutic targets for multiple immunotherapy targets as well as tumor-targeted mAbs. Expression of the human FcRs seems to match the expected expression pattern (Smith et al. 2012). Of course, while these mice are an invaluable tool, they are still subject to the inherent weaknesses of mouse tumor models, where immune infiltrates and specifically immune cells expressing FcRs are different from human tumors.

3.2 Antibodies Targeting Myeloid Cell Populations

In addition to depletion of Treg cells, other suppressive immune cell types can be removed by mAb treatment. One example being explored clinically is CSF1R, which targets myeloid cells thought to restrain T cell responses to tumors. CSF1 is a growth factor required for the survival of these cells, and the cell type can be targeted with either small molecules that inhibit the kinase function of the receptor or mAbs that prevent binding of CSF1R to its ligands CSF1 and IL-34. The mAb cabiralizumab, which is in clinical testing in combination with nivolumab, is an IgG4, and is not thought to require effector function for its activity. A mouse surrogate (mIgG1) of this mAb has been shown to have antitumor activity in mouse models and to specifically reduce M2 macrophages at the tumor site. While both the surrogate and human mAbs employ Fcs that should not induce ADCC, a mAb that does induce ADCC may be more effective at eliminating this cell type. Inhibiting CSF1R signaling is also being investigated using the humanized Ab, emactuzumab, which blocks the dimerization interface of CSF1R and is in ongoing Phase 1 clinical trials in combination with atezolizumab.

Myeloid-derived suppressor cells (MDSC) are another suppressive cell type that could be targeted with depleting mAbs. Using a Ly6G mAb, Clavijo et al. showed depletion of Ly6G+ , Ly6Cint myeloid cells that they classified as granulocytic MDSCs (Clavijo et al. 2017). This depletion of MDSCs combined with CTLA-4 treatment resulted in complete rejection of the MOC1 tumor model, but had no effect on tumor growth in the MOC2 model. The authors speculated that this difference in responses was due to the lack of antigen and T-cell infiltrate in the MOC2 model. While this data suggests targeting MDSCs could be a powerful therapeutic strategy in combination with other immunotherapies, the lack of specific markers of MDSCs in humans complicates the application of this strategy to cancer patients. As tumor-infiltrating macrophages may also be critical effector cells for cytotoxic and checkpoint control antibodies, a highly specific targeting of MDSCs is of critical importance (Lehmann et al. 2017; Simpson et al. 2013).

A mAb can also be used to target multiple cell populations at once, based on expression of its target. Daratumumab, a human IgG1 mAb specific for CD38, has been approved for the treatment of multiple myeloma. CD38 is a promising target for MM as it is highly expressed on these tumor cells. It is also highly expressed on a variety of immune suppressive cell populations such as granulocytic MDSCs,

Bregs, and a highly suppressive fraction of human Tregs. Daratumumab has been shown to mediate ADCC of these populations in vitro and in the case of Bregs and CD38-expressing Tregs, patients treated with daratumumab have reduced numbers of these cell types, consistent with ADCC (Krejcik et al. 2016).

3.3 Antagonist Antibodies

While a depleting mAb targeting CTLA-4 has been shown to confer superior antitumor activity to a mAb that does not engage FcR, this is not true for all T-cell inhibitory receptors. In contrast to CTLA-4 and most costimulatory receptors, PD-1 is expressed at higher levels on CD8 T cells in the tumor than in Tregs. Targeting PD-1 with a depleting mAb isotype can preferentially deplete CD8 cells and result in an abrogated antitumor response in comparison with a non-depleting isotype (Dahan et al. 2015). Therefore, the expression pattern of the mAb target on Tregs and T effector cells is likely to determine the strategy that should be employed to target the receptor.

3.4 Agonist Antibodies

Antibodies can be used to initiate signaling through a receptor as well as to block binding to the receptor's ligand. In some cases, such as the CD28 superagonist, this may occur simply through soluble binding of the mAb to the receptor, but signaling may also be improved by Ab binding to FcR bearing cells (Bartholomaeus et al, 2014). More commonly there is a requirement for the mAb to bind to another surface in order to achieve the higher valency required. In vitro, this is often accomplished by binding the mAb to plastic in the form of a plate or bead. The mAb then mediates the formation of clustered receptors necessary for signaling. In vivo, it is thought that FcRs can mediate this higher valency and allow mAbs to work as agonists even if they cannot trigger signaling without crosslinking.

Agonist mAbs have been most well studied in the context of the TNF receptor superfamily. TNFRs require the formation of higher-order clusters to signal, and hence, often require mAbs to be crosslinked by FcR to mediate signaling in vivo. CD40 is expressed on antigen presenting cells and is critical in promoting immune activation by inducing expression of costimulatory ligands on APCs. The activation of CD40 can be studied by using a DEC205-based vaccination system. Using this system Li and Ravetch (Li and Ravetch 2011) demonstrated that the inhibitory Fc receptor, FcγRIIb was required for CD40 agonist activity, and that mAbs that preferentially bind to activating receptors such as mIgG2a or mAbs that did not bind FcR such as the mIgG1 D265A mutant, did not confer agonist activity. Similar results were found in human FcR transgenic mice, where a human IgG1 S267E mutation significantly enhanced agonist activity compared to the human IgG1 mAb or an FcR nonbinder (N297A) (Li and Ravetch 2013). Importantly, the requirement for preferential FcγRIIb binding was also confirmed in mouse tumor models, where a mIgG1 mAb against CD40 was more efficacious than mIgG2a or mIgG1 D265A mAbs. Separate work from White et al. using a different vaccination system also confirmed the requirement for FcγRIIb interactions while utilizing a different CD40 agonist mAb (White et al. 2011).

In addition to CD40, the importance of FcγRIIb binding has also been demonstrated for other agonistic mAbs such as Fas, DR4, and DR5. Anti-Fas antibodies were shown to have significantly less hepatotoxicity in FcγRIIb KO mice than in wild-type mice, indicating that the inhibitory FcR is necessary for Fas agonism (Xu et al. 2003). For DR4, the mIgG1 isotype had higher antitumor efficacy in the Colo205 mouse tumor model than the mIgG2a version and similar results were seen in multiple tumor models for a DR5 mAb (Chuntharapai et al. 2001). In the case of DR5, the S267E mutation was able to enhance activity compared to the human IgG1 in the MC38 and 4T1 tumor models when these expressed human FcγRIIb in place of the mouse homolog (Li and Ravetch 2012). Together these data confirm the role of CD32B in mediating agonist signaling for targets expressed on APCs or tumors themselves.

Extrapolating this data to T cell costimulatory targets is more complicated. As mentioned earlier, mAbs against GITR and OX-40 are more active when formatted to engage with activating receptors. Similar data have been observed for mAbs against ICOS (Engelhardt et al. unpublished observations). These observations are driven primarily by the depletion of Tregs at the tumor site and likely are not representative of which mAb formats induce the best agonist signal through the receptor in question. Antibodies against another TNFRSF member, CD27, have also been shown to have antitumor activity, in this case in human CD27 transgenic mice (wild-type mouse FcR). This activity was dependent on FcR binding, as the human IgG1 mAb had activity while the N297S version did not (He et al. 2013). These results do not indicate whether activity is due to a depleting or agonistic mechanism (Wasiuk et al. 2017). For most if not all mAbs directed against costimulatory receptors expressed on Tregs and effector T cells, activity in mouse tumor models will be highest with depleting isotypes rather than those that preferentially engage the inhibitory receptor. This hierarchy may not translate to humans though, as it is unclear that Treg depletion occurs as readily in patients as in mice. If depletion is not a relevant mechanism in humans or in cases where an agonist is potentially being combined with another agent that depletes Tregs, it may be advantageous to have a mAb that is optimized for agonist function via crosslinking by CD32B. It is possible that binding to activating Fc receptors may lead to depletion in some circumstances and agonism in others further complicating the interpretation of the data from mouse tumor models.

Most T-cell agonist programs that have moved to the clinic so far have utilized human IgG1 mAbs or in the case of urelumab an IgG4 mAb. These programs have thus shown limited antitumor efficacy as monotherapy, with no agonist mAb having gained approval to date. It may be that a superior CD32B binding mutant would have more activity than what has been observed so far.

4 Conclusions

The use of monoclonal mAbs in cancer treatment allows for the targeting of proteins and cell populations with high specificity. An improved understanding of the interactions between mAb Fc regions and FcγRs has led to the design of therapeutics that lead to distinct effects after the binding of the mAb to its antigen. Antibodies can be optimized for specific purposes as shown in Fig. 1. Initial therapeutics targeted the cancer cells themselves and relied on FcR⁺ cells as effectors to kill the cancer cells through ADCC or ADCP. Human IgG1 mAbs were first used to mediate this killing, but advances in the field of mAb engineering have led to the use of nonfucosylated or Fc mutated mAbs that enhance the interactions leading to ADCC or ADCP. With the advent of immunotherapy, mAbs have also been used to alter the immune response to tumors, that is, target, and eradicate inhibitory immune cells by ADCC or ADCP, thereby allowing other immune cells to recognize and kill the cancer cells. It has long been known that mAbs can stimulate signaling through a receptor and mimic ligand binding. This often requires clustering of the receptors on the cell surface that can be accomplished in vivo by the binding of the mAb Fc to FcRs. In multiple systems, this is most efficiently accomplished by binding to the inhibitory receptor CD32B and this binding can be enhanced and made more selective to CD32B through mutation to the Fc region. Finally, mAbs can be used to block binding of a particular receptor or ligand on an immune cell. In this case, an absence of binding to FcR is often preferable and can be accomplished by choosing an isotype with low affinity for FcRs such as IgG4 or including Fc mutations that further reduce FcR binding.

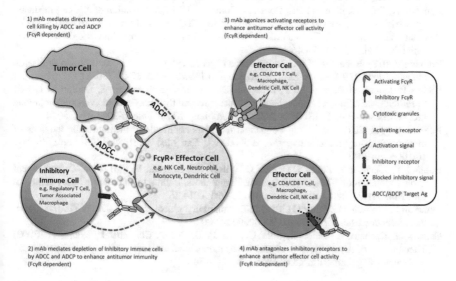

Fig. 1 Critical role of FcγRs in promoting antibody-mediated tumor immunity

Antibodies are powerful tools for treating cancer patients, and understanding the role of FcγRs in the function of therapeutic mAbs will enable the design of more powerful therapeutics.

Acknowledgements The authors thank Catherine A. Bolger for her review and editing, and Alan J. Korman for his critical reading and insightful perspective on this chapter.

References

Abès R et al (2010) Long-lasting antitumor protection by anti-CD20 antibody through cellular immune response. Blood 116(6):926–934

Albanell J, Baselga J (1999) Trastuzumab, a humanized anti-HER2 monoclonal antibody, for the treatment of breast cancer Drugs Today (Barc) 35:931–946

Amiri-Kordestani L et al. (2014a) FDA approval: ado-trastuzumab emtansine for the treatment of patients with HER2-positive metastatic breast cancer Clin Cancer Res 20:4436–4441 https://doi.org/10.1158/1078-0432.ccr-14-0012

Amiri-Kordestani L et al. (2014b) First FDA approval of neoadjuvant therapy for breast cancer: pertuzumab for the treatment of patients with HER2-positive breast cancer Clin Cancer Res 20:5359–5364 https://doi.org/10.1158/1078-0432.ccr-14-1268

Barnhart BC, Quigley M (2017) Role of Fc-FcgammaR interactions in the antitumor activity of therapeutic antibodies. Immunol Cell Biol 95:340–346. https://doi.org/10.1038/icb.2016.121

Bartholomaeus P et al (2014) Cell contact-dependent priming and Fc interaction with CD32 + immune cells contribute to the TGN1412-triggered cytokine response. J Immunol 192:2091–2098. https://doi.org/10.4049/jimmunol.1302461

Bezman NA et al (2017) PD-1 blockade enhances elotuzumab efficacy in mouse tumor models blood advances 1:753–765

Blair HA (2018) Atezolizumab: A Review in Previously Treated Advanced Non-Small. Cell Lung Cancer Target Oncol 13:399–407. https://doi.org/10.1007/s11523-018-0570-5

Bouchon A, Cella M, Grierson HL, Cohen JI, Colonna M (2001) Activation of NK cell-mediated cytotoxicity by a SAP-independent receptor of the CD2 family. J Immunol 167:5517–5521

Boulianne GL, Hozumi N, Shulman MJ (1984) Production of functional chimaeric mouse/human antibody. Nature 312:643–646

Bruhns P (2012) Properties of mouse and human IgG receptors and their contribution to disease models. Blood 119:5640–5649. https://doi.org/10.1182/blood-2012-01-380121

Bruhns P, Iannascoli B, England P, Mancardi DA, Fernandez N, Jorieux S, Daeron M (2009) Specificity and affinity of human Fcgamma receptors and their polymorphic variants for human IgG subclasses. Blood 113:3716–3725. https://doi.org/10.1182/blood-2008-09-179754

Bulliard Y et al (2013) Activating Fc gamma receptors contribute to the antitumor activities of immunoregulatory receptor-targeting antibodies. J Exp Med 210:1685–1693. https://doi.org/10.1084/jem.20130573

Bulliard Y, Jolicoeur R, Zhang J, Dranoff G, Wilson NS, Brogdon JL (2014) OX40 engagement depletes intratumoral Tregs via activating FcgammaRs, leading to antitumor efficacy Immunol Cell Biol 92:475–480. https://doi.org/10.1038/icb.2014.26

Cameron F, Whiteside G, Perry C (2011) Ipilimumab: first global approval. Drugs 71:1093–1104. https://doi.org/10.2165/11594010-000000000-00000

Cartron G, Dacheux L, Salles G, Solal-Celigny P, Bardos P, Colombat P, Watier H (2002) Therapeutic activity of humanized anti-CD20 monoclonal antibody and polymorphism in IgG Fc receptor FcgammaRIIIa gene. Blood 99:754–758

Cheney CM et al (2014) Ocaratuzumab, an Fc-engineered antibody demonstrates enhanced antibody-dependent cell-mediated cytotoxicity in chronic lymphocytic leukemia. MAbs 6:749–755. https://doi.org/10.4161/mabs.28282

Chuntharapai A et al (2001) Isotype-dependent inhibition of tumor growth in vivo by monoclonal antibodies to death receptor 4. J Immunol 166:4891–4898

Clavijo PE et al (2017) Resistance to CTLA-4 checkpoint inhibition reversed through selective elimination of granulocytic myeloid cells. Oncotarget 8:55804–55820. https://doi.org/10.18632/oncotarget.18437

Clynes R (2006) Antitumor antibodies in the treatment of cancer: Fc receptors link opsonic antibody with cellular immunity. Hematol Oncol Clin North Am 20:585–612. https://doi.org/10.1016/j.hoc.2006.02.010

Clynes RA, Towers TL, Presta LG, Ravetch JV (2000) Inhibitory Fc receptors modulate in vivo cytotoxicity against tumor targets. Nat Med 6:443–446. https://doi.org/10.1038/74704

Coe D, Begom S, Addey C, White M, Dyson J, Chai JG (2010) Depletion of regulatory T cells by anti-GITR mAb as a novel mechanism for cancer immunotherapy. Cancer Immunol Immunother 59:1367–1377. https://doi.org/10.1007/s00262-010-0866-5

Collins SM et al (2013) Elotuzumab directly enhances NK cell cytotoxicity against myeloma via CS1 ligation: evidence for augmented NK cell function complementing ADCC. Cancer Immunol Immunother 62:1841–1849. https://doi.org/10.1007/s00262-013-1493-8

Dahan R, Sega E, Engelhardt J, Selby M, Korman AJ, Ravetch JV (2015) FcgammaRs modulate the anti-tumor activity of antibodies targeting the PD-1/PD-L1 axis. Cancer Cell 28:285–295. https://doi.org/10.1016/j.ccell.2015.08.004

Dhillon S (2015) Dinutuximab: first global approval. Drugs 75:923–927. https://doi.org/10.1007/s40265-015-0399-5

Dienstmann R, Tabernero J (2010) Necitumumab, a fully human IgG1 mAb directed against the EGFR for the potential treatment of cancer Curr Opin Investig. Drugs 11:1434–1441

DiLillo DJ, Ravetch JV (2015) Fc-receptor interactions regulate both cytotoxic and immunomodulatory therapeutic antibody effector functions cancer. Immunol Res 3:704–713. https://doi.org/10.1158/2326-6066.CIR-15-0120

Ferrara N, LeCouter J, Lin R, Peale F (2004) EG-VEGF and Bv8: a novel family of tissue-restricted angiogenic factors. Biochim Biophys Acta 1654:69–78. https://doi.org/10.1016/j.bbcan.2003.07.001

Forero-Torres A et al (2012) Results of a phase 1 study of AME-133v (LY2469298), an Fc-engineered humanized monoclonal anti-CD20 antibody, in FcgammaRIIIa-genotyped patients with previously treated follicular lymphoma. Clin Cancer Res 18:1395–1403. https://doi.org/10.1158/1078-0432.ccr-11-0850

Gbadamosi M, Meshinchi S, Lamba JK (2018) Gemtuzumab ozogamicin for treatment of newly diagnosed CD33-positive acute myeloid leukemia. Future Oncol. https://doi.org/10.2217/fon-2018-0325

Giusti RM, Shastri KA, Cohen MH, Keegan P, Pazdur R (2007) FDA drug approval summary: panitumumab (Vectibix). Oncologist 12:577–583. https://doi.org/10.1634/theoncologist.12-5-577

Goede V et al (2014) Obinutuzumab plus chlorambucil in patients with CLL and coexisting conditions. N Engl J Med 370:1101–1110. https://doi.org/10.1056/NEJMoa1313984

Goldberg RM (2005) Cetuximab. Nat Rev Drug Discov Suppl:S10–11

Grillo-Lopez AJ (2002) Zevalin: the first radioimmunotherapy approved for the treatment of lymphoma.Expert Rev Anticancer Ther 2:485–493. https://doi.org/10.1586/14737140.2.5.485

He LZ et al (2013) Agonist anti-human CD27 monoclonal antibody induces T cell activation and tumor immunity in human CD27-transgenic mice. J Immunol 191:4174–4183. https://doi.org/10.4049/jimmunol.1300409

Hsi ED et al (2008) CS1, a potential new therapeutic antibody target for the treatment of multiple myeloma. Clin Cancer Res 14:2775–2784. https://doi.org/10.1158/1078-0432.ccr-07-4246

Jakobovits A (1998) The long-awaited magic bullets: therapeutic human monoclonal antibodies from transgenic mice. Expert Opin Investig Drugs 7:607–614. https://doi.org/10.1517/13543784.7.4.607

Jakubowiak AJ et al (2016) Cost-effectiveness of adding carfilzomib to lenalidomide and dexamethasone in relapsed multiple myeloma from a US perspective J. Med Econ 19:1061–1074. https://doi.org/10.1080/13696998.2016.1194278

Jones PT, Dear PH, Foote J, Neuberger MS, Winter G (1986) Replacing the complementarity-determining regions in a human antibody with those from a mouse. Nature 321:522–525. https://doi.org/10.1038/321522a0

Kazandjian D et al (2016) FDA approval summary: Nivolumab for the treatment of metastatic non-small cell lung cancer with progression on or after platinum-based chemotherapy. Oncologist 21:634–642. https://doi.org/10.1634/theoncologist.2015-0507

Kerr DJ (2004) Targeting angiogenesis in cancer: clinical development of bevacizumab. Nat Clin Pract Oncol 1:39–43. https://doi.org/10.1038/ncponc0026

Kim ES (2017) Avelumab: first global approval. Drugs 77:929–937. https://doi.org/10.1007/s40265-017-0749-6

Kim YH et al (2018) Mogamulizumab versus vorinostat in previously treated cutaneous T-cell lymphoma (MAVORIC): an international, open-label, randomised, controlled phase 3 trial. Lancet Oncol. https://doi.org/10.1016/s1470-2045(18)30379-6

Klein C et al (2013) Epitope interactions of monoclonal antibodies targeting CD20 and their relationship to functional properties. MAbs 5:22–33. https://doi.org/10.4161/mabs.22771

Ko K et al (2005) Treatment of advanced tumors with agonistic anti-GITR mAb and its effects on tumor-infiltrating Foxp3 + CD25 + CD4 + regulatory. T cells J Exp Med 202:885–891. https://doi.org/10.1084/jem.20050940

Köhler G, Milstein C (1975) Continuous cultures of fused cells secreting antibody of predefined specificity. Nature 256:495

Kohrt HE et al (2012) Combination strategies to enhance antitumor ADCC. Immunotherapy 4:511–527. https://doi.org/10.2217/imt.12.38

Krejcik J et al (2016) Daratumumab depletes CD38 + immune regulatory cells, promotes T-cell expansion, and skews T-cell repertoire in multiple myeloma. Blood 128:384–394

Leach DR, Krummel MF, Allison JP (1996) Enhancement of antitumor immunity by CTLA-4 blockade. Science 271:1734–1736

Lehmann B et al (2017) Tumor location determines tissue-specific recruitment of tumor-associated macrophages and antibody-dependent immunotherapy response. Sci Immunol 2.pii: eaah6413. https://doi.org/10.1126/sciimmunol.aah6413

Li F, Ravetch JV (2011) Inhibitory Fcgamma receptor engagement drives adjuvant and anti-tumor activities of agonistic CD40 antibodies. Science 333:1030–1034. https://doi.org/10.1126/science.1206954

Li F, Ravetch JV (2012) Apoptotic and antitumor activity of death receptor antibodies require inhibitory Fcgamma receptor engagement. Proc Natl Acad Sci U S A 109:10966–10971. https://doi.org/10.1073/pnas.1208698109

Li F, Ravetch JV (2013) Antitumor activities of agonistic anti-TNFR antibodies require differential FcgammaRIIB coengagement in vivo. Proc Natl Acad Sci U S A 110:19501–19506. https://doi.org/10.1073/pnas.1319502110

Lonial S et al (2015) Elotuzumab Therapy for Relapsed or Refractory Multiple Myeloma. N Engl J Med 373:621–631. https://doi.org/10.1056/NEJMoa1505654

Lu D et al (2003) Tailoring in vitro selection for a picomolar affinity human antibody directed against vascular endothelial growth factor receptor 2 for enhanced neutralizing activity. J Biol Chem 278:43496–43507. https://doi.org/10.1074/jbc.m307742200

Lundin J et al (1998) CAMPATH-1H monoclonal antibody in therapy for previously treated low-grade non-Hodgkin's lymphomas: a phase II multicenter study. European Study Group of CAMPATH-1H Treatment in Low-Grade Non-Hodgkin's Lymphoma. J Clin Oncol 16:3257–3263. https://doi.org/10.1200/jco.1998.16.10.3257

Mahne AE et al (2017) Dual roles for regulatory T-cell depletion and costimulatory signaling in agonistic GITR targeting for tumor immunotherapy. Cancer Res 77:1108–1118. https://doi.org/10.1158/0008-5472.CAN-16-0797

Maloney DG et al (1997) IDEC-C2B8 (Rituximab) anti-CD20 monoclonal antibody therapy in patients with relapsed low-grade non-Hodgkin's lymphoma. Blood 90:2188–2195

Markham A (2016) Elotuzumab: first global approval drugs 76:397–403. https://doi.org/10.1007/s40265-016-0540-0

McKeage K (2016) Daratumumab: first global approval. Drugs 76:275–281. https://doi.org/10.1007/s40265-015-0536-1

Morrison SL, Johnson MJ, Herzenberg LA, Oi VT (1984) Chimeric human antibody molecules: mouse antigen-binding domains with human constant region domains. Proc Natl Acad Sci U S A 81:6851–6855

Nimmerjahn F, Ravetch JV (2005) Divergent immunoglobulin g subclass activity through selective Fc receptor binding. Science 310:1510–1512

Ogura M et al (2014) Multicenter phase II study of mogamulizumab (KW-0761), a defucosylated anti-cc chemokine receptor 4 antibody, in patients with relapsed peripheral T-cell lymphoma and cutaneous T-cell lymphoma. J Clin Oncol 32:1157–1163. https://doi.org/10.1200/jco.2013.52.0924

Osterborg A et al (2016) Phase III, randomized study of ofatumumab versus physicians' choice of therapy and standard versus extended-length ofatumumab in patients with bulky fludarabine-refractory chronic lymphocytic leukemia Leuk. Lymphoma 57:2037–2046. https://doi.org/10.3109/10428194.2015.1122783

Overdijk MB et al (2015) Antibody-mediated phagocytosis contributes to the anti-tumor activity of the therapeutic antibody daratumumab in lymphoma and multiple myeloma. In: MAbs, vol 2. Taylor & Francis, pp 311–320

Park KU et al (2010) Gene expression analysis of ex vivo expanded and freshly isolated NK cells from cancer patients. J Immunother 33:945–955. https://doi.org/10.1097/CJI.0b013e3181f71b81

Pierpont TM, Limper CB, Richards KL (2018) Past, present, and future of rituximab—the world's first oncology monoclonal antibody therapy. Front Oncol 8:163. https://doi.org/10.3389/fonc.2018.00163

Plitas G et al (2016) Regulatory T cells exhibit distinct features in human breast cancer. Immunity 45:1122–1134. https://doi.org/10.1016/j.immuni.2016.10.032

Poole RM (2014) Pembrolizumab: first global approval. Drugs 74:1973–1981. https://doi.org/10.1007/s40265-014-0314-5

Poole RM, Vaidya A (2014) Ramucirumab: first global approval. Drugs 74:1047–1058. https://doi.org/10.1007/s40265-014-0244-2

Ravetch JV, Lanier LL (2000) Immune inhibitory receptors Science 290:84–89

Salles G et al. (2012) Phase 1 study results of the type II glycoengineered humanized anti-CD20 monoclonal antibody obinutuzumab (GA101) in B-cell lymphoma patients. Blood 119:5126–5132. https://doi.org/10.1182/blood-2012-01-404368

Selby MJ, Engelhardt JJ, Quigley M, Henning KA, Chen T, Srinivasan M, Korman AJ (2013) Anti-CTLA-4 antibodies of IgG2a isotype enhance antitumor activity through reduction of intratumoral regulatory T cells. Cancer Immunol Res 1:32–42. https://doi.org/10.1158/2326-6066.cir-13-0013

Serna-Gallegos TR, La-Fargue CJ, Tewari KS (2018) The ecstacy of gold: patent expirations for Trastuzumab, Bevacizumab, Rituximab, and Cetuximab Recent Pat. Biotechnol 12:101–112. https://doi.org/10.2174/1872208311666171122152131

Shields RL et al (2002) Lack of fucose on human IgG1 N-linked oligosaccharide improves binding to human Fcgamma RIII and antibody-dependent cellular toxicity. J Biol Chem 277:26733–26740. https://doi.org/10.1074/jbc.m202069200

Shirley M (2017) Olaratumab: first global approval. Drugs 77:107–112. https://doi.org/10.1007/s40265-016-0680-2

Simpson TR et al (2013) Fc-dependent depletion of tumor-infiltrating regulatory T cells co-defines the efficacy of anti-CTLA-4 therapy against melanoma. J Exp Med 210:1695–1710. https://doi.org/10.1084/jem.20130579

Smith P, DiLillo DJ, Bournazos S, Li F, Ravetch JV (2012) Mouse model recapitulating human Fcgamma receptor structural and functional diversity. Proc Natl Acad Sci U S A 109:6181–6186. https://doi.org/10.1073/pnas.1203954109

Stagg J, Divisekera U, Duret H, Sparwasser T, Teng MW, Darcy PK, Smyth MJ (2011) CD73-deficient mice have increased antitumor immunity and are resistant to experimental metastasis. Cancer Res 71:2892–2900. https://doi.org/10.1158/0008-5472.can-10-4246

Syed YY (2017) Durvalumab: first global approval. Drugs 77:1369–1376. https://doi.org/10.1007/s40265-017-0782-5

Tai YT et al (2008) Anti-CS1 humanized monoclonal antibody HuLuc63 inhibits myeloma cell adhesion and induces antibody-dependent cellular cytotoxicity in the bone marrow milieu Blood 112:1329–1337. https://doi.org/10.1182/blood-2007-08-107292

Tam SH et al (2017) Functional, biophysical, and structural characterization of human IgG1 and IgG4 variants with ablated immune functionality. Antibodies 6:1–34

Taylor LD et al (1992) A transgenic mouse that expresses a diversity of human sequence heavy and light chain immunoglobulins. Nucleic Acids Res 20:6287–6295

Tobinai K et al (2011) Phase I study of LY2469298, an Fc-engineered humanized anti-CD20 antibody, in patients with relapsed or refractory follicular lymphoma. Cancer Sci 102:432–438. https://doi.org/10.1111/j.1349-7006.2010.01809.x

Tuaillon N, Taylor LD, Lonberg N, Tucker PW, Capra JD (1993) Human immunoglobulin heavy-chain minilocus recombination in transgenic mice: gene-segment use in mu and gamma transcripts. Proc Natl Acad Sci U S A 90:3720–3724

Tvito A, Rowe JM (2017) Inotuzumab ozogamicin for the treatment of acute lymphoblastic leukemia. Expert Opin Biol Ther 17:1557–1564. https://doi.org/10.1080/14712598.2017.1387244

van der Veer MS et al (2011) The therapeutic human CD38 antibody daratumumab improves the anti-myeloma effect of newly emerging multi-drug therapies. Blood Cancer J 1:e41

Wasiuk A et al (2017) CD27-mediated regulatory T cell depletion and effector T cell costimulation both contribute to antitumor efficacy. J Immunol 199:4110–4123. https://doi.org/10.4049/jimmunol.1700606

Weiner LM, Dhodapkar MV, Ferrone S (2009) Monoclonal antibodies for cancer immunotherapy. Lancet 373:1033–1040. https://doi.org/10.1016/S0140-6736(09)60251-8

Weng WK, Levy R (2003) Two immunoglobulin G fragment C receptor polymorphisms independently predict response to rituximab in patients with follicular lymphoma. J Clin Oncol 21:3940–3947. https://doi.org/10.1200/JCO.2003.05.013

White AL et al (2011) Interaction with FcgammaRIIB is critical for the agonistic activity of anti-CD40 monoclonal antibody. J Immunol 187:1754–1763. https://doi.org/10.4049/jimmunol.1101135

Xu Y et al (2003) Fc gamma Rs modulate cytotoxicity of anti-Fas antibodies: implications for agonistic antibody-based therapeutics. J Immunol 171:562–568

Yamane-Ohnuki N, Satoh M (2009) Production of therapeutic antibodies with controlled fucosylation. MAbs 1:230–236

Younes A, Bartlett NL, Leonard JP, Kennedy DA, Lynch CM, Sievers EL, Forero-Torres A (2010) Brentuximab vedotin (SGN-35) for relapsed CD30-positive lymphomas. N Engl J Med 363:1812–1821. https://doi.org/10.1056/nejmoa1002965

Anti-inflammatory Activity of IgG-Fc

Christopher Beneduce, Elma Kurtagic and Carlos J. Bosques

Contents

Abstract Over 80 different autoimmune disorders have been identified. A common denominator across most of these disorders is the presence of pathogenic autoantibodies. The pathogenic and inflammatory nature of antibodies is well accepted, and over the last three decades, evidence in humans and rodent models has revealed that antibodies can induce anti-inflammatory activities. The discovery of the relationship between immunoglobulin G (IgG) glycovariants and disease activity in autoimmune patients has provided insight into the structural and functional characteristics of IgG associated with its pro- and anti-inflammatory activity. In this chapter, we discuss evidence of the anti-inflammatory nature of IgG and the mechanisms by which this activity is exerted. Current clinical evidence of this anti-inflammatory activity is also discussed.

C. Beneduce · E. Kurtagic · C. J. Bosques (✉)
Research Department, Momenta Pharmaceuticals, Cambridge, USA
e-mail: cbosques@momentapharma.com

Current Topics in Microbiology and Immunology (2019) 423: 35–62
https://doi.org/10.1007/82_2019_148
© Springer Nature Switzerland AG 2019
Published online: 22 February 2019

1   Introduction

The role of immunoglobulin G (IgG) in the pathogenesis of many autoimmune disorders such as systemic lupus erythematosus (SLE), myasthenia gravis, immune thrombocytopenia, and many other diseases is well defined. Autoantibodies can form immune complexes with their cognate antigen and trigger inflammatory processes through their interaction with cellular Fc gamma receptors (FcγRs) and complement. It is now understood that IgG can also have anti-inflammatory activities. The pro- and anti-inflammatory activity of IgG can be modulated by different properties of the Ig such as the IgG subclass, glycosylation, and valency. The composition of the Fc domain, although it is considered the invariant region of the IgG molecule, is highly heterogeneous. In addition to the four distinct sub-classes of human IgG (IgG1, IgG2, IgG3, and IgG4), the Fc domain exhibits additional diversity in individual allotypes and glycosylation states. Furthermore, IgG can form complexes with target ligands, antigens, cells, or particles, leading to different degrees of Fc valency. The combination of subclass, allotype, glycosy-lation, and valency leads to a substantial amount of heterogeneity in Fc structure (Arnold et al. 2007; Vidarsson et al. 2014), which can influence the interaction of IgG with its receptors and ultimately influence its function. Effector functions of human IgG are carried out by complement and by the FcγRs. Humans express several activating FcγRs, including FcγRI, FcγIIa, FcγIIc, FcγIIIa, and the lone inhibitory FcγRIIb. Activating FcγRs signal via a highly conserved immunore-ceptor tyrosine-based activation motif. FcγRIIa and FcγRIIc intrinsically express this motif in their γ chain, whereas FcγRI and FcγRIIIa rely on the common FcR γ chain (γ_2) to trigger activating signals. In contrast, FcγRIIb contains an immunoreceptor tyrosine-based inhibition motif (ITIM) in its α chain. Activating FcγRs are commonly found on myeloid cells, dendritic cells (DCs), natural killer (NK) cells, and neutrophils. The inhibitory FcγRIIb is typically expressed together with activating FcγRs. B cells are a notable exception as they express FcγRIIb only and do not express activating FcγRs.

FcγRs exhibit different affinities for IgG subclasses. FcγRI can bind all human IgG subclasses with relatively high affinity, with the exception of IgG2. FcγRI has the unique ability to interact with monomeric IgG. FcγRIIa, the most widely expressed receptor, can bind all IgG subclasses, and it is the only FcγR to bind to IgG2a. IgG3 binding affinity is highest for FcγRIIa, followed by IgG1, with weak but measurable binding affinity to IgG2 and IgG4. Variants of FcγRIIa have been described to modulate affinity for IgG2a, with the 131R variant having higher affinity than the 131H variant. IgG binding affinity to FcγRIIb is weak for all subclasses, and affinity for IgG2 is the lowest. FcγRIIIa, which binds all subclasses, has two well-described variants: FV158 and V158. V158 has a greatly increased affinity for all IgG subclasses and a particularly high affinity for IgG3. FcγRIIIb, which is mostly expressed on neutrophils, binds IgG1 and IgG3, with little binding to IgG2 and IgG4. FcγRIIIb also has two allotypic variants, denoted NA1 and NA2.

The NA1 allotype exhibits higher binding affinity to IgG1 and IgG3 subclasses and an increased ability to phagocytose IgG1- and IgG3-opsonized particles (Bruhns et al. 2009; Vidarsson et al. 2014).

Overall, human and mouse FcγRs, with the exception of FcγRI, have low affinity for monomeric IgG. They preferentially bind IgG in the form of immune complexes. Immune complex multivalent binding results in multimeric clustering of FcγRs and signaling cascades that involves spleen tyrosine kinase (SYK), phospholipase C (PLC), and calcium release, ultimately resulting in activation of the ERK/AKT pathways. Depending on the cell type, signaling via activating FcγRs results in cellular proliferation, generation of reactive oxygen species (ROS), antibody-dependent cellular phagocytosis (ADCP), antibody-dependent cellular cytotoxicity (ADCC), and cytokine production. Conversely, immune complex interaction with FcγRIIb results in quelling of the proinflammatory activities of the activating FcγRs. This process is mediated by the FcγRIIb ITIM domain and the SH2-containing inositol phosphatase (SHIP). It is well accepted that FcγRIIb counterbalances signals triggered by the activating FcγRs in cells of the innate immune system and modulates signaling of the B-cell receptor (BCR) on B cells. In 2000, Clynes et al. demonstrated that FcγRIIb could modulate the in vivo ADCC activity of the anti-CD20 antibody rituximab (Clynes et al. 2000). Co-ligation of the inhibitory FcγRIIb with activating FcγRs was shown to inhibit the activation and maturation of dendritic cells and inhibit FcγRIIa-mediated cytokine release (Boruchov et al. 2005). Co-ligation of FcγRIIb and the B-cell receptor on B cells is known to inhibit BCR-mediated signaling in a SHIP-mediated manner resulting in reduced B-cell activation and proliferation (Chu et al. 2008; Heyman 2003; Kiener et al. 1997; Ono et al. 1997).

IgG glycosylation is crucial in modulating the in vivo activity of IgG. All IgG molecules contain a single conserved N-linked glycosylation site (Asn-297) in each of the constant heavy two (C_H2) domains, critical for maintaining their proinflammatory and anti-inflammatory effector functions (Arnold et al. 2007; Schwab and Nimmerjahn 2013). The sugar moiety attached to Asp-297 predominantly consists of an octasaccharide biantennary structure, composed of four N-acetylglucosamines (GlcNac), three mannoses, and one fucose, which may contain terminal galactose or sialic acid residues. These glycans help maintain the quaternary structure and the stability of the Fc (Mimura et al. 2000, 2001) and are vitally involved in FcγR binding through maintenance of an open conformation of the two heavy chains (Jefferis and Lund 2002; Sondermann et al. 2001). Deglycosylated IgG has been shown to lose nearly all significant FcγR and C1q binding affinity (Nose and Wigzell 1983). Evidence that deglycosylated IgG antibodies are unable to mediate in vivo inflammatory responses accounts for the requirement of the glycans for FcγR binding (Nimmerjahn and Ravetch 2006). Fc glycans are critical for maintaining both the proinflammatory and the anti-inflammatory effector functions of IgG (Arnold et al. 2007). Branching fucose residues at the core of the biantennary glycan have had a significant effect on the IgG-Fc binding affinity for FcγRIIIa, with afucosylated IgG having a much higher affinity for the receptor

(Ferrara et al. 2011; Houde et al. 2010; Nimmerjahn and Ravetch 2005; Shields et al. 2002; Shinkawa et al. 2003).

The terminal sugar residues in the IgG-Fc can consist of N-acetylglucosamine, galactose, or sialic acid. Sialylated IgG glycoforms have decreased binding affinity to several FcRs (Kaneko et al. 2006b) and can adversely impact IgG-Fc proinflammatory function (Scallon et al. 2007). In addition, changes in Fc glycosylation have been shown to modulate complement-dependent cytotoxicity where increasing amounts of terminal galactose increase the binding affinity of the complement C1q to the IgG-Fc (Raju 2008).

2 Clinical Relevance of IgG Glycosylation in Humans

A common feature of most autoimmune diseases is the formation of immune complexes between pathogenic IgG autoantibodies and cognate antigens. These immune complexes activate inflammatory effector cells expressing FcγRs and the complement cascade, contributing to tissue damage. Apart from antibody isotype and subclass, the function of autoantibodies is in part modulated by their Fc N-linked glycans. An example of the role of autoantibody glycosylation in disease pathogenicity was provided by Lood et al. The authors demonstrated that enzymatic deglycosylation of SLE immune complexes in vitro abolished their proinflammatory properties (Lood et al. 2012). Immune complex deglycosylation eliminated several important proinflammatory properties of immune complexes that are important in SLE pathogenesis: FcγR-mediated phagocytosis, interferon alfa (IFN-α) production, polymorphonuclear leukocytes chemotaxis, and classical pathway of complement activation. Furthermore, deglycosylation of immune complexes from SLE patients also had a direct effect on the molecular structure of immune complexes, causing decreased immune complex size, emphasizing the crucial role of Fc glycans for immune complex-mediated pathological signals.

In contrast to studies that link hypoglycosylation of immune complexes and the resulting loss of proinflammatory activity, results of other studies have shown that glycoforms that specifically lack terminal sialic acid or galactose residues (G0 glycoforms) might have increased proinflammatory activity. Original observations from the 1980s showed that IgG glycosylation differs in patients with rheumatoid arthritis, with decreased Fc galactosylation and sialylation compared with normal individuals (Parekh et al. 1985). Since then, a difference in the glycosylation profile of total IgG has been reported in patients with various other autoimmune diseases, including SLE, inflammatory bowel disease, myasthenia gravis, ankylosing spondylitis, primary Sjögren's syndrome, psoriatic arthritis, and multiple sclerosis (Dube et al. 1990; Selman et al. 2011; Trbojevic Akmacic et al. 2015; Vuckovic et al. 2015; Watson et al. 1999; Wuhrer et al. 2015a). In addition to their association with autoimmune diseases, agalactosylated polyclonal antibodies are associated with increased inflammation in infectious diseases such as HIV (Ackerman et al. 2013). Besides the evidence of disparate IgG glycans in different autoimmune disease, therapeutic treatments and changes in the physiologic state can also result in differential IgG glycosylation. Namely, treatment of patients with rheumatoid arthritis with methotrexate can lead to increased levels of IgG galactosylation and hence a decrease in the abundance of agalactosylated IgG-G0 glycoforms (Pasek et al. 2006)). Furthermore, IgG-G0 glycoforms were decreased in women with rheumatoid arthritis during pregnancy, correlating with reduced incidence of flares (Rook et al. 1991; van de Geijn et al. 2009). Additional evidence suggests that serum levels of IgG-G0 glycans increase shortly before the onset of disease in patients with rheumatoid arthritis (Rombouts et al. 2015). Presumably, a window of time for initiation of preventative treatment could be estimated based on the abundance of G0 glycoforms. More recently, it was shown that treatment with estrogen in postmenopausal women with rheumatoid arthritis significantly increased IgG-Fc sialylation (Engdahl et al. 2018).

One of the best examples of specific monosaccharide residue impacting the proinflammatory activity of IgG is the core N-linked glycan fucose. Glycoforms lacking core fucose residues have been shown to have altered affinities for individual FcγRs (Shields et al. 2002). Defucosylation of IgG resulted in 10- to 50-fold enhanced affinity for mouse FcγRIV and human FcγRIII (Ferrara et al. 2011; Nimmerjahn and Ravetch 2005; Shields et al. 2002; Shinkawa et al. 2003). Consequently, defucosylation in the Fc domain of antibodies leads to increased antibody-dependent cell-mediated cytotoxic activity (Ferrara et al. 2011; Nechansky et al. 2007). Furthermore, results of a series of studies showed enhanced cytotoxic and phagocytic activity in mouse tumor and autoimmune models using these IgG glycovariants, indicating the importance of glycoengineering of antibodies for improved clinical effectiveness. In fact, therapeutic antibodies that lack fucose residues have shown enhanced tumor killing in cancer patients and have been approved as therapy for different B-cell cancers. Although there is abundant evidence of strongly increased IgG-G0 glycoforms in patients during active autoimmune disease, fucosylated IgG seems to remain stable during inflammation and vaccination in mice and humans (Kao et al. 2017; Kemna et al. 2017; Rombouts et al. 2015; Scherer et al. 2010; Selman et al. 2011; Sjowall et al. 2015). However, there are recent reports of disparate fucosylation levels of alloantibodies in hemolytic disease of the fetus or newborn (HDFN) (Kapur et al. 2014a) and fetal and neonatal alloimmune thrombocytopenia (FNAIT) (Kapur et al. 2014b; Sonneveld et al. 2016; Wuhrer et al. 2009), diseases that arise because of maternal alloimmunization against paternally inherited red blood cell antigen Rh-D or platelets, respectively. These alloantibodies are transported across the placenta and result in severe fetal anemia or thrombocytopenia. Systematical analysis of IgG-derived glycopeptides from 70 anti-D alloantibodies from pregnant women revealed a decrease in Fc-fucosylation (Kapur et al. 2014b), which correlated significantly with FcγRIIIa-mediated ADCC. Furthermore, low Fc-fucosylation correlated with severe fetal anemia (Sonneveld et al. 2017). Thus, even though IgG fucosylation levels are generally stable during various autoimmune diseases, there is a strong correlation between antibody fucosylation and disease severity during pregnancy, and those antibodies play an active role in disease pathogenicity.

The anti-inflammatory activity of sialylated IgG is evident in patients as several studies have reported changes in IgG sialylation levels during inflammation and presence of autoimmune diseases. For instance, patients with rheumatoid arthritis, granulomatosis with polyangiitis (GPA), antiphospholipid syndrome (APS), vasculitis, and SLE have low serum levels of IgG or low autoantibody sialylation (Espy et al. 2011; Fickentscher et al. 2015; Kemna et al. 2017; Vuckovic et al. 2015; Wuhrer et al. 2015b). One particular study reported significantly higher sialylation of IgG recognizing anti-2-glycoprotein 1 autoantibodies (2GP1-IgG) isolated from the sera of healthy children and asymptomatic adults compared with that of patients with clinically apparent anti-phospholipid syndrome (APS) (Fickentscher et al. 2015). Another group demonstrated that histone IgG autoantibodies purified from SLE patients displayed significantly lower sialylation than total IgG of the same patients, suggesting that the SLE utoantibodies contain proinflammatory activities (Magorivska et al. 2016). In patients with GPA, characterized by the presence of antineutrophil cytoplasmic antibodies (ANCA) against proteinase-3 (PR3), pathogenic proteinase 3 autoantibodies are less sialylated in patients with active Wegener's vasculitis (GPA) than in those with inactive disease (Espy et al. 2011). The authors further demonstrated that purified anti-PR3 antibodies from patients with active disease were proinflammatory, and enzymatic desialylation of anti-PR3 antibodies from patients with inactive disease restored pathogenic activity (Espy et al. 2011). This study provided direct evidence of the importance of autoantibody sialylation as it pertains to the modulation of antibody activity in an autoimmune disease. Furthermore, it was shown that total IgG-Fc of patients with severe ANCA-associated vasculitis (AAV) exhibits lower levels of galactosylation, sialylation, and bisecting N-acetylglucosamine (GlcNAc) compared with healthy controls (Wuhrer et al. 2015b). This finding was more pronounced for PR3-ANCA antibodies than with total IgG.

Potential use of circulating levels of sialylated IgG as a disease biomarker is noteworthy. Serum levels of sialylated IgG have decreased shortly before disease relapses, similar to galactosylated IgG, showing promise as a predictive biomarker (Kemna et al. 2017; Rombouts et al. 2015). Patients with GPA exhibited low galactosylation or low sialylation of total IgG1 and were highly prone to relapse after ANCA increase. When relapsing patients were examined, total IgG1 sialylation decreased from the time of the PR3-ANCA increase to the relapse, while the glycosylation profile remained similar in nonrelapsing patients (Kemna et al. 2017). An intriguing observation is that low sialylation was observed in total IgG1 and not in antigen-specific PR3, and low sialylation of total IgG1 predicted disease reactivation in patients with GPA who experienced ANCA increase during follow-up. Along the same lines, studies have shown a reduction in sialylation of IgG in chronic inflammatory demyelinating polyneuropathy (CIDP), and this reduction correlated with clinical severity of the disease. This observation implies potential use of sialylated IgG as a biomarker to monitor disease severity in CIDP (Wong et al. 2016). Restoring serum antibody sialylation correlated with treatment response in patients with Guillain-Barre syndrome (Fokkink et al. 2014) and Kawasaki disease (Ogata et al. 2013), where lower sialylation of endogenous IgG predicted resistance to therapy (Ogata et al. 2013). Taken together all the evidence summarized above, monitoring of sialylated IgG antibodies during different phases of an antibody-mediated disease may have diagnostic and prognostic potential and could help optimize the treatment of patients with autoimmune diseases.

3 Role of Sialylation in the Anti-inflammatory Activity of Intravenous Immunoglobulin

Despite the decade-long clinical effectiveness of intravenous immunoglobulin (IVIg) in treating inflammatory and autoimmune diseases, the mechanism of action of IVIg has remained enigmatic. IVIg is effective in a wide range of diseases in which many mechanisms of the underlying disease are not well understood, further complicating the understanding of all the details of IVIg anti-inflammatory mechanisms. Moreover, the fact that IgG can form many different binding interactions through antigen binding and Fc domains adds to the complexity. Many hypotheses have been proposed to explain the reasons for the seemingly paradoxical activity of high-dose IVIg. One theory attributes IVIg activity to the polyclonal binding specificities that are encoded in the variable region of the administered antibodies, which in turn may counteract the activity of autoantibodies and inflammatory mediators, as shown in toxic epidermal necrolysis (Viard et al. 1998). However, intact IVIg and its Fc fragments have almost identical activity in many animal models (Bruhns et al. 2003; Kaneko et al. 2006b; Samuelsson et al. 2001) and in the clinical treatment of idiopathic thrombocytopenic purpura (ITP) (Debre et al. 1993). Therefore, the emergence of evidence attributing the anti-inflammatory activity of IVIg to its Fc portion has promoted further investigation and focus on Fc-mediated mechanisms. For example, saturation of the neonatal FcRn—leading to increased catabolism of pathogenic autoantibodies—has been proposed as one of the primary mechanisms of IVIg (Akilesh 2004; Hansen and Balthasar 2002; Li et al. 2005). However, the evidence to support this proposal is limited because of the difficulty in experimentally modeling FcRn dependence since removing FcRn in mice results in rapid clearance of exogenous autoantibodies and in strongly reduced serum IgG levels (Vaccaro et al. 2005).

Another proposed mechanism is the saturation of activating FcγRs and prevention of pathogenic autoantibodies from triggering FcγRs activation, thereby limiting their pathogenic potential. For example, monoclonal antibodies that block activating FcγRs have mimicked the anti-inflammatory properties of IVIg (Siragam et al. 2006).

Furthermore, the dimeric and aggregate fraction in IVIg may facilitate multivalent avid interactions with low-affinity FcγRs and inhibit their activation by pathogenic immune complexes. Indeed, it has been experimentally shown that the protective effects of IVIg can be mimicked by the injection of opsonized red blood cells or by soluble immune complexes (Siragam et al. 2005). More recently, recombinant multivalent Fc molecules with avid binding to low-affinity FcγRs have also demonstrated similar anti-inflammatory properties to IVIg (Zuercher et al. 2016).

Another proposed mechanism of action for IVIg is the induction of anti-inflammatory activities by altering the relative surface expression of activating and inhibiting FcγRs in favor of the inhibitory FcγRIIb, thereby increasing the signal threshold necessary to activate immune cells (Anthony et al. 2011; Schwab and Nimmerjahn 2013). As it was long postulated, immune complex-induced inflammatory responses are regulated by the relative expression of activating versus inhibitory FcγRs on effector cells, dictating the threshold of immune complex-induced inflammation (Ravetch and Clynes 1998). In fact, it was demonstrated in animal models of ITP, autoimmune hemolytic anemia, rheumatoid arthritis, and nephrotoxic nephritis that the ability of IVIg to protect mice from pathogenic IgG was dependent on FcγRIIb (Akilesh 2004; Crow et al. 2003; Huang et al. 2010; Kaneko et al. 2006a, b; Samuelsson et al. 2001). Similarly, results of several studies showed that FcγRIIb is upregulated on innate immune effector cells and B cells after IVIg treatment in mice (Bruhns et al. 2003; Kaneko et al. 2006b; Samuelsson et al. 2001). Furthermore, this was confirmed in patients with CIDP, in whom FcγRIIb expression levels on B cells were impaired. Interestingly, FcγRIIb protein expression was upregulated on monocytes and B cells after clinically effective IVIg therapy (Tackenberg et al. 2009).

Given all the evidence of anti-inflammatory activities of high-dose IVIg treatment, it has become apparent that the preparations of IVIg from normal human donors indeed contain a small fraction of active therapeutic that is not necessarily an oligomer. The first study to strongly correlate Fc glycosylation and biological activity of IVIg was reported by Kaneko 2006 and was later substantiated by results of several studies in a variety of animal models of autoimmune disease (Anthony et al. 2008a; Kaneko et al. 2006b; Schwab et al. 2012; Tackenberg et al. 2009). Biochemical characterizations of IVIg preparations that display anti-inflammatory activities in animal models pointed to the absolute requirement for the Fc fragment and its N-linked biantennary glycan attached at the Asn-297 (Kaneko et al. 2006b). The authors demonstrated that highly sialylated forms of monoclonal mouse IgG have reduced affinity for FcγR and cytotoxic function. Furthermore, the anti-inflammatory activity of IVIg was shown to be mediated mainly by a small fraction of antibodies containing terminal sialic acid on their oligosaccharide structures. Interestingly, a stronger protective effect of the IVIg fraction enriched for sialic acid was also shown. Enzymatic removal of the sialic acid residues abrogated the anti-inflammatory activity of IVIg in a mouse model of rheumatoid arthritis. These studies also showed that sialylation of the IVIg Fc fragment was sufficient for anti-inflammatory activities (Kaneko et al. 2006b).

4 Impact of Sialylation on IgG Structure and Anti-inflammatory Activity

Work by Ravetch and others has helped shed light on how different IgG glycoforms can impact the anti-inflammatory activity of IgG (Anthony et al. 2008a; Crow et al. 2003; Kaneko et al. 2006b; Samuelsson et al. 2001; Schwab et al. 2014). Structural studies revealed that the IgG-Fc may adopt "open" or "closed" confirmations depending on the glycosylation state. For example, the Fc glycans at position 297 have been shown to contribute to an "open" conformation of the IgG-Fc in which the C_H2 domains are separated by larger distances than in deglycosylated Fc structures (Krapp et al. 2003). Conversely, the deglycosylated IgG displays a conformation in which the C_H2 region adopts a "closed" state (Feige et al. 2009). More recent crystallographic work highlighted a higher conformational heterogeneity of the C_H2 domain in sialylated IgG-Fc protein fragments. The specific interactions between the N297 glycans and the amino acid backbone of the C_H2 domain are interrupted upon terminal sialylation, which can help explain these conformational changes (Ahmed et al. 2014). It was demonstrated how a specific point mutation (F241A) in the Fc domain could recapitulate the flexibility seen with sialylated glycoforms (Fiebiger et al. 2015). These structural characterizations may help explain how earlier studies showed that highly sialylated IgG significantly reduced affinity for the canonical FcγRs (Kaneko et al. 2006b). These changes in Fc structure could also help explain how highly sialylated IgG shows reduced ability to induce effector functions such as ADCC (Scallon et al. 2007). Some findings suggest otherwise, where highly sialylated species were unchanged or only slightly reduced in their ability to bind activating FcγRs (Li et al. 2017; Subedi and Barb 2016). One study suggested that Fc sialylation can also modulate an antibody Fab binding to its cognate antigen via altered flexibility of the hinge region. This reduced flexibility may restrict the antibody to monovalent Fab binding to its target, thus reducing its apparent affinity (Scallon et al. 2007).

In addition to modulating classic FcγR binding, Fc sialylation can increase IgG affinity for type II FcRs including DC-SIGN and CD23 (Anthony et al. 2008a; Sondermann et al. 2013). DC-SIGN (Dendritic Cell-Specific ICAM3-Grabbing Non-Integrin), a C-type Lectin, is found most commonly on the surface of dendritic cells and macrophages. It has been shown to recognize bacterial and viral pathogen-associated molecular patterns and is involved in HIV pathogenesis (Gringhuis et al. 2014; Mogensen et al. 2010). The murine analog of DC-SIGN, SIGN-R1, was shown to be necessary for the anti-inflammatory activity of IVIg in the KBX/N mouse model of arthritis (Anthony et al. 2008a). The activity of IVIg could be restored in SIGN-R1$^{-/-}$ mice when reconstituted with human DC-SIGN. Although SIGN-R1 is not expressed on dendritic cells in mice, it is highly expressed on a population of CSF1-dependent macrophages that reside in the marginal zone of the spleen (Anthony et al. 2008a; Schwab and Nimmerjahn 2013). In 2003, Bruhns et al. had shown that CSF1-dependent macrophages were responsible for the in vivo activity of IVIg. Studies using op/op mice deficient in

CSF1 implied that IVIg induced FcγRIIb upregulation through an indirect mechanism. It was suggested that IVIg may interact with CSF1-dependent regulatory cells, which in turn leads to the upregulated expression of FcγRIIb on separate CSF1-independent effector cells (Bruhns et al. 2003). Work by Anthony and colleagues in 2011 presented a unified hypothesis to help reconcile IVIg requirements for Fc sialylation, FcγRIIb, and SIGN-R1 for its anti-inflammatory activity in various models of autoimmunity. Using the KBX/N model, the researchers showed how IVIg, via interaction with DC-SIGN-positive splenic myeloid cells, caused the release of interleukin (IL) 33, which in turn induced the production of IL-4. IL-4 was then shown to be involved in upregulation of FcγRIIb on effector macrophages, thereby increasing their threshold of immune complex-mediated activation. Mice deficient in the IL-4 receptor were refractory to IVIg therapy, and systemic administration of IL-33 or IL-4 suppressed serum-induced arthritis. The source of IL-4 in these mice was determined to be basophils, which produce Il-4 in response to IL-33 stimulation (Anthony et al. 2011). Figure 1 summarizes the mechanism proposed by Ravetch and coworkers to explain the requirement of Fc sialylation for the anti-inflammatory activity of IVIg. This study laid the groundwork for understanding how intrinsic sialylated IgG could help maintain immune homeostasis. Both IVIg and sialylated IVIg, but not unsialylated IVIg, upregulated IL-33 mRNA in spleens of treated animals, and sialylated IVIg was more potent in a model of antiganglioside antibody-mediated inhibition of axon regeneration, supporting the previously proposed mechanisms (Zhang et al. 2016).

The question of whether this particular anti-inflammatory mechanism of IVIg plays a role in human patients is unclear given that marginal zone macrophages are absent in the human spleen (Steiniger et al. 1997). Furthermore, some ITP patients who underwent splenectomies still respond to IVIg therapy (Cines and Bussel 2005), and studies in ITP mouse models demonstrated that the inhibitory effects of sialylated IVIg were not impaired after splenectomy (Leontyev et al. 2012; Schwab et al. 2012), suggesting a potential different pathway in humans or in specific disease settings. Schwab et al. showed that, in addition to IVIg activity not being impaired in mice that underwent splenectomy, neither the activating FcγRs FcγRI and FcγRIII nor the cytokines requiring the common cytokine γ chain or the IL-33 receptor were involved in this anti-inflammatory pathway suppressing murine ITP. However, IVIg activity was still fully dependent on the terminal sialic acid and SIGN-R1, most likely on a cell type outside the spleen (Schwab et al. 2012). Perhaps IVIg mechanisms might be different depending on whether IVIg is administered before induction of autoimmune disease or inflammation (such is the case in the majority of the reported studies) versus IVIg administration during acute autoimmune disease. Recent studies addressed this question and showed that, under therapeutic conditions in mouse models of ITP, inflammatory arthritis, and the autoimmune skin blistering disease epidermolysis bullosa acquisita, IVIg activity was fully dependent on IgG sialylation and FcγRIIb. However, SIGN-R1 was only partially required, suggesting that select pathways may be involved in mediating IVIg activity when treating established autoimmune disease (Schwab et al. 2014).

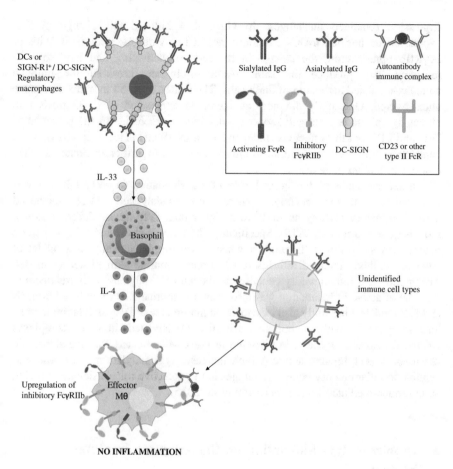

Fig. 1 Schematic representation of mechanism proposed by Ravetch and coworkers to explain the requirement of Fc sialylation for IVIg anti-inflammatory activity (Anthony et al. 2008b; Bruhns et al. 2003; Sondermann et al. 2013; Maamary et al. 2017) Ig, immunoglobulin; IL, interleukin

However, the exact pathways during patient treatment with IVIg were not addressed in those studies.

Some recent studies have helped elucidate whether this T-helper type 2 (TH2) cascade occurs in human patients treated with IVIg. IVIg studies in humans have shown that high-dose IVIg does induce IL-33 and IL-4 in patients with various inflammatory myopathies (Schwab et al. 2014; Tjon et al. 2014). Similar results with IL-33 were seen in IVIg-treated patients with Guillain-Barre syndrome, but this was not a predictor of therapeutic success (Maddur et al. 2017). The study by Tjon et al. aimed to address the variations between mice and humans and demonstrated that the IL-33 TH2 pathway by which IVIg inhibits myeloid cells in mice may also be used in humans but with slight variations (Tjon et al. 2014). Namely, instead of FcγRIIb upregulation, FcγRIIa was downregulated on circulating myeloid dendritic cells (mDCs) from IVIg-treated patients while FcγRIIb expression remained unchanged. In vitro, IL-4 induced this change in FcR expression on purified mDCs. Although not in line with observations in mice of FcγRIIb upregulation, the change in the ratio of activating and inhibitory Fc receptors may produce the same result of higher threshold for immune complex-mediated activation of these cells. The source of IL-33 in humans remains undiscovered. One study did note an increased expression of IL-33 mRNA in human lymph node cells and monocyte-derived macrophages in the presence of IVIg and LPS, but this effect was independent of DC-SIGN (Tjon et al. 2014). More controlled studies with IVIg in the clinic are necessary to further elucidate this TH2 cascade in human patients.

Further evidence of the crucial role of Fc sialylation in IVIg efficacy was demonstrated more recently, where tetra-Fc-sialylated IVIg enhanced anti-inflammatory activity up to 10-fold higher than IVIg across different animal models (Washburn et al. 2015). Specifically, the tetra-Fc-sialylated IVIg was more potent than the parent IVIg product when dosed prophylactically in a model of collagen antibody-induced arthritis (CAIA) and a murine skin blistering model. Therapeutic anti-inflammatory benefit with the tetra-Fc-sialylated IVIg treatment at the time of active inflammation was also shown in murine K/BxN-induced arthritis and ITP models. One study also extended the importance of IVIg sialylation in bone loss in patients with rheumatoid arthritis. Desialylated immune complexes enhanced osteoclastogenesis in vivo and in vitro. Mice treated with the sialic acid precursor N-acetylmannosamine, which increases IgG sialylation, were less susceptible to inflammatory bone loss, suggesting a protective role of sialylated IgG in autoimmune-mediated bone loss (Harre et al. 2015).

5   Impact of IgG Sialylation on the Adaptive Immune System

The observation that T cells, purified from IVIg-treated nonimmunodeficient children, significantly suppressed pokeweed mitogen-induced B-cell and T-cell proliferation provided the first indication that IVIg could modulate the adaptive immune system (Durandy et al. 1981). In vitro experiments from the same study showed that this modulation of T-cell suppressor activity was Fc-mediated. As a follow-up, other publications noted the increase in the suppressive activities of T cells after IVIg treatment in ITP and AIDs (Delfraissy et al. 1985; Gupta et al. 1986). Since then, IVIg has been shown to increase the number of circulating T-regulatory cells (Tregs) in Guillain-Barre syndrome, SLE, eosinophilic granulomatosis with polyangiitis (Churg–Strass syndrome), Kawasaki disease, and a peripheral neuropathy known as mononeuritis multiplex, among others (Barreto et al. 2009; Burns et al. 2013; Chi et al. 2007; Tsurikisawa et al. 2012, 2014). Various mechanisms have been proposed to explain how IVIg can modulate suppressor T-cell function and frequency. One possible Fc-specific mechanism was described in patients with Kawasaki disease where IVIg treatment induces the expansion of IL-10-producing Tregs with TCR specificity for peptides derived from IgG-Fc (Franco et al. 2014). It was later shown by the same group that these Tregs could be activated in a major histocompatibility complex (MHC)-restricted manner by autologous IgG-positive B cells in the absence of exogenous Fc. Interestingly, these Fc-specific Tregs were present in IVIg-treated patients with Kawasaki disease patients and in healthy adult donors (Burns and Franco 2015).

Successful induction of Treg responses requires signals in the form of soluble cytokines and costimulatory molecules, typically provided by professional antigen-presenting cells (APCs) such as dendritic cells, macrophages, and B cells. IVIg has been shown to modulate dendritic cell function in various ways. Decreased expression of costimulatory markers such as CD80/86 and MHC class II on IVIg-exposed dendritic cells results in decreased capacity for these cells to drive lymphocyte proliferation (Bayry et al. 2003; Kaufman et al. 2011; Qian et al. 2011). In addition, IVIg has been shown to induce dendritic cell production of inhibitory and anti-inflammatory cytokines such as IL-10 (Bayry et al. 2003; Massoud et al. 2012; Ohkuma et al. 2007; Ramakrishna et al. 2011). Work from De Groot et al. and others has suggested a role for dendritic cells in the presentation of IgG-derived T-cell epitopes known as "Tregitopes," which contain peptides from both the Fab and the Fc fragments of IgG (De Groot et al. 2008; Ephrem et al. 2008). In the DeGroot model, dendritic cells uptake IVIg and process it for loading of peptides onto MHC class II, allowing for activation and expansion of Tregs.

Specifically, it is debatable which receptors on APC IVIg might interact with. The obvious candidates are the type I and type II FcRs. FcγRIIa and FcγRIIb are found on subsets of dendritic cells and macrophages. Activating FcγRs on dendritic cells are necessary for successful treatment of ITP (Siragam et al. 2006). In this model, the researchers hypothesized that IVIg formed immune complexes in vivo, which acted on dendritic cells, thus priming their regulatory activity. The investigators developed an adoptive transfer model in which isolated dendritic cells were primed with IVIg in vitro and subsequently transferred to mice with active ITP. The IVIg-primed dendritic cells were able to ameliorate ITP in these mice even when the dendritic cells lacked FcγRIIb. Interestingly, the IVIg-primed dendritic cells were unable to ameliorate ITP when the host mouse lacked FcγRIIb expression. This suggests that the IVIg-dendritic cell interaction is independent of FcγRIIb, but the receptor was still necessary for later phases of IVIg action (Siragam et al. 2006). Substantiating this finding, IVIg and immune complexes containing sialylated IgGs were able to inhibit the LPS-induced maturation of bone marrow-derived dendritic cells independently of FcγRIIb (Oefner et al. 2012). One study, using a similar model of adoptive transfer, showed that IVIg-primed bone marrow-derived dendritic cells (BMDCs) could induce Treg activity and be used to successfully treat mice with ovalbumin-induced airway hyperresponsiveness (AHR), but IVIg effectiveness was not disturbed when the BMDCs lacked activating FcRs (Massoud et al. 2014). In this same study, the researchers found that IVIg ability to ameliorate AHR was almost entirely dependent on the dendritic cell immunoreceptor (DCIR). DCIR is an ITIM-bearing C-type lectin receptor found mostly on monocyte and dendritic cell populations (Kanazawa 2007). Massoud et al. showed that Treg induction in AHR by IVIg was dependent on Cd11c-positive dendritic cells, but they were unable to detect expression of the type II Fc receptor SIGN-R1 on these cells. Instead, they observed DCIR-dependent binding of sialylated IVIg glycoforms and DCIR-dependent induction of Tregs.

The type II FcγR SIGN-R1 is expressed mainly on macrophages in mice, whereas DC-SIGN is expressed on myeloid and plasmacytoid dendritic cells and on some macrophages in humans. Fieberger et al. reported that IVIg required DC-SIGN/ SIGN-R1 in amelioration of both T-cell-mediated and autoantibody-mediated diseases (Fiebiger et al. 2015). They demonstrated that a single-point mutation at F241A in recombinant Fc, even when lacking terminal sialic acid, conferred the same protections as sialylated Fc in the KBX/N model of arthritis. IVIg and the F241A Fc but not unsialylated IVIg were shown to expand FoxP3+ Tregs in KBX/N-naive and KBX/N-challenged mice. Both IVIg and F241A Fc were also able to expand Treg and suppress T-cell-mediated autoimmunity in the experimental autoimmune encephalitis (EAE) model in a SIGN-R1/DC-SIGN-dependent manner. Finally, inhibition of IL-33 signaling abrogated IVIg and F241A Fc ability to induce Treg and suppress inflammation, lending more support to this group's original proposal of TH2 cytokine cascade as the underlying cause of sialylated IVIg anti-inflammatory activity (Fiebiger et al. 2015). Do DCIR and DC-SIGN/SIGN-R1 operate independently of one another to induce Treg expansion and activity in response to sialylated IVIg treatment? More studies are necessary to address how these receptors and the cells upon which they are expressed mediate IVIg ability to induce Treg.

Modulation of T-cell responses in models of delayed-type hypersensitivity (DTH) by sialylated IgGs was reported by Oefner et al. in 2012. DTH reactions require antigen uptake, processing, and presentation to T-helper cells, which in turn produce proinflammatory cytokines, resulting in tissue inflammation. In the Oefner et al. model of ovalbumin-induced DTH injection of sialic-rich ovalbumin-specific IgG, but not antibodies of different antigen specificity, they were able to suppress DTH responses. Sialylated immune complexes were shown to inhibit dendritic cell maturation in an FcγRIIb-independent manner, which could explain this inhibition of DTH. Although both the antigen specificity and the FcγRIIb independence of the sialylated IgG ability to inhibit DTH in this model are in contrast to reports of IVIg-mediated suppression of antibody responses, modulation of T-cell responses is still a common denominator (Oefner et al. 2012).

6   Modulation of Autoantibody Pathogenicity by Sialylation

Although most understanding of the anti-inflammatory activity of IgG comes from experience with IVIg, more recent studies have helped translate the IVIg findings to antigen-specific IgG autoantibodies. One particular study elegantly demonstrated how antigen-specific antibodies, when sialylated, could be used not only to reverse autoantibody-mediated inflammation, but also to prevent development of disease. Ohmi et al. showed that genetic knockdown of mSt6gal1, a glycotransferase responsible for transferring sialic acid to galactose, specifically in activated B cells resulted in higher incidence and earlier development of collagen-induced arthritis (CIA), along with more severe joint swelling in the affected mice (Ohmi et al. 2016). Enforcing sialylation of the ACC4 monoclonal antibody used to stimulate collagen antibody-induced arthritis in DBA-1 mice abolished the development of disease in all mice. Using the CIA model, the researchers demonstrated that, after immunization with bovine type II collagen, treatment of mice with sialylated ACPAs resulted in delayed incidence of disease and less severe joint swelling. In addition, treatment of CIA with the sialylated ACPAs resulted in in vivo production of sialylated anti-type II collagen antibodies (Ohmi et al. 2016).

The anti-inflammatory activity of specific sialylated antibodies was also shown in models of IgG- and IgE-mediated anaphylaxis. Although allergen-induced anaphylaxis is mostly induced by IgE, it can also be mediated by IgG produced in response to high levels of allergen. In the presence of excess allergen, these IgGs have the potential to activate complement and FcγRs on various effector cells, leading to anaphylaxis. However, allergen-specific IgG antibodies, which are often induced by allergen-specific immunotherapies (AITs), have also been shown to inhibit IgE-mediated anaphylaxis (Burton et al. 2014; Strait et al. 2006). This is accomplished through a combination of allergen masking and FcγRIIb engagement. Just as FcγRIIb can mediate inhibition of the activating FcγRs, cross-linking of FcγRIIb with the IgE receptor FcεRI on basophils and mast cells can prevent activation of these cells and, thus, limit release of various proinflammatory mediators implicated in allergen-induced anaphylaxis (Strait et al. 2006). In line with these observations, TNP-specific IgG1 antibodies were unable to inhibit anti-TNP IgE-mediated anaphylaxis in response to challenge with TNP-Ova in FcγRIIb$^{-/-}$ mice (Epp et al. 2018). In a similar model, it was shown that desialylated and degalactosylated IgG1 and IgG2 anti-TNP antibodies induce more severe anaphylaxis in response to challenge with TNP-Ova. In contrast, sialylated anti-TNP IgG1 effectively inhibited TNP-Ova-induced anaphylaxis. This effect was dependent on FcγRIIb and SIGN-R1. In humans, AITs typically elicit allergen-specific IgG4 antibodies. These studies used mouse IgG1 antibodies, which resemble human IgG4 in their complement and classical FcγR binding (Epp et al. 2018). This study highlights the possibility that AIT protocols that induce sialylated IgGs might limit IgG-mediated anaphylaxis in patients exposed to high doses of allergen. To this end, the researchers showed that immunization of mice with Ova in the adjuvant monophosphoryl lipid A, which was recently approved for AIT, resulted in production of sialylated and galactosylated IgG1 and IgG2, which were limited in their ability to induce IgG-mediated anaphylaxis (Epp et al. 2018).

Immune complexes formed by autoantibodies and their cognate antigens have also been shown, in certain scenarios, to mediate anti-inflammatory processes. As discussed in previous sections, it is clear that IgG glycosylation changes during disease progression and sialylation is often correlated with low disease activity (Espy et al. 2011; Fickentscher et al. 2015; Kemna et al. 2017; Parekh et al. 1985; Pasek et al. 2006). In vitro analysis of these sialylated autoantibodies and immune complexes has helped shed light on some of the mechanisms by which inflammation is controlled by antibody glycosylation. In the case of SLE, antihistone antibodies isolated from patients were shown to be mostly asialylated and were able to mediate efficient phagocytosis when used to opsonize necrotic cells, a hallmark of SLE pathology (Magorivska et al. 2016). Sialylated autoantibodies isolated from these patients were less effective at mediated neutrophil phagocytosis and switched inflammatory cytokine production form IL-6/IL-8 to IL-1b/TNF-α (Magorivska et al. 2016). Earlier studies had shown similar results in anti-PR3 antibodies isolated from patients with active GPA (Espy et al. 2011). The authors demonstrated that autoantibodies isolated from patients with active disease, exhibiting low sialic acid content, induced a greater oxidative burst in neutrophils than those from patients with quiescent disease. Enzymatic desialylation of anti-PR3 antibodies from those patients with inactive GPA resulted in restoration of pathogenic activity (Espy et al. 2011). In rheumatoid arthritis, anticitrullinated protein antibodies (ACPAs) are known to induce innate cell-mediated inflammation in and around joints, resulting in bone destruction (Kurowska et al. 2017). These ACPAs can contain less Fc sialylation than other circulating IgGs (Ohmi et al. 2016; Rombouts et al. 2015; Scherer et al. 2010). Studies in mice have shown that these ACPAs promote osteoclastogenesis, resulting in bone resorption. In following up on these findings, it was found that desialylated immune complexes increased osteoclastogenesis in an FcγRII- and FcγRIII-mediated manner. Furthermore, treatment of CIA in mice with ManNAc, a precursor to sialic acid, resulted in increased sialylation of circulating IgG1, delayed induction of arthritis, and reduced severity of the disease (Harre et al. 2015).

Taken together, these studies show that, when sialylated, antigen-specific autoantibodies possess anti-inflammatory properties. The results of these studies have large implications for the development of antigen-specific immunotherapies for autoimmune disorders whose autoantigens are well defined. In line with this notion, a recent study took a different approach and attempted to sialylate antibodies in vivo as a means of making them anti-inflammatory. The researchers investigated how administration of B4GALT1 and ST6GAL1, glycotransferases that transfer galactose and sialic acid, respectively, modulated autoantibody function in murine models of arthritis. Coadministration of these enzymes before the transfer of K/BxN sera resulted in marked reduction in inflammation similar to that seen with IVIg treatment (Pagan et al. 2018). This treatment was also effective in a model of Goodpasture syndrome, in which coadministration of the enzymes markedly inhibited kidney disease. Keeping with the aforementioned TH2 anti-inflammatory cascade initiated by sialylated IgG, in vivo sialylation and the resulting anti-inflammatory activity achieved with these enzymes had a strict requirement of FcγRIIb and SIGN-R1 (Pagan et al. 2018).

7 Anti-inflammatory Activity of Multivalent IgG-Fc

Immune complexes formed by the interaction between autoantibodies and self-antigens are drivers of pathogenicity in many inflammatory and autoimmune diseases. The inflammatory mechanisms are driven by activation of complement pathways or through FcγR-mediated cellular activation. Briefly, all FcγRs except FcγRI bind Fc domains with low affinity. For effective cell activation, FcγRs require immune complexes for their aggregation, resulting in ultimate activation of downstream signaling. Inhibition of these pathways through competition with IgG-Fc molecules with high valency has been explored as a potential therapeutic alternative. In fact, commercial IVIg preparations may contain a small fraction of higher-order IgG structures in the form of dimers and aggregates, which presumably are important for the anti-inflammatory activities of IVIg (Teeling et al. 2001).

All these observations have stimulated the development of recombinant oligomeric Fc proteins as potential replacement for IVIg (Zuercher et al. 2016). Figure 2 provides an overview of multimeric Fc drug candidates currently in preclinical or clinical studies. Stradomer (GL-2045) generated by Gliknik/Pfizer (Gliknik. Gliknik pipeline products. http://www.gliknik.com/pipeline/) is a drug candidate consisting of a mixture of heterogenous IgG-Fc oligomeric structures. In particular, stradomers are fully recombinant fusion proteins composed of murine IgG2a-Fc hinge and either the human IgG2H or isoleucine zipper multimerization domains, existing as homodimers and as a high percentage of covalently linked highly

Drug Candidate	Description	Institution	Structure
Stradomer GL2045	Heterogeneous IgG-Fc multimer with IgG2 hinge	Gliknik/Pfizer	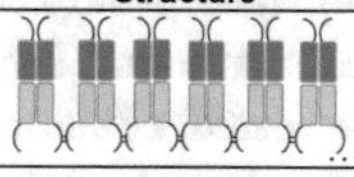
Fc3Y or M230/CSL730	3 IgG1-Fc domains	Momenta Pharmaceuticals/CSL	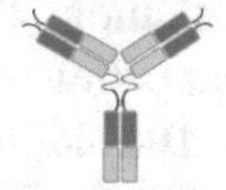
Hexamers	HexaGard: Hexameric IgG-Fc with IgM tailpiece with L309/H310L	Liverpool School of Tropical Medicine	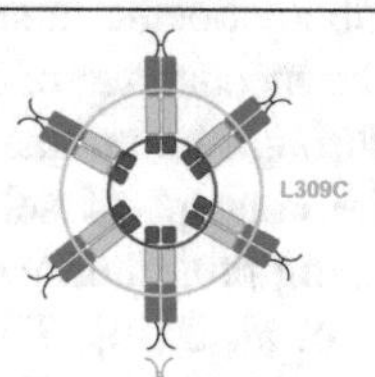
	CSL777: Hexameric IgG-Fc with IgM tailpiece with L309C	CSL	
	γ1 or γ4: IgG1 or IgG4 Hexameric Fc	UCB	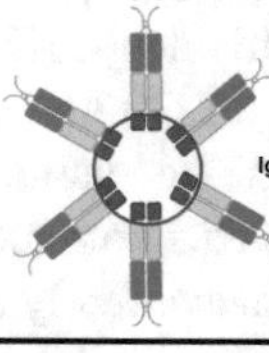

Fig. 2 Summary of multimeric Fc drug candidates being explored as anti-inflammatory agents. Ig, immunoglobulin

ordered multimers (Jain et al. 2012). Stradomers prevented the onset of ITP and ameliorated symptoms in other autoimmune disease models, including collagen-induced arthritis (Jain et al. 2012), experimental autoimmune neuritis (Niknami et al. 2013), and autoimmune myasthenia gravis (Thiruppathi et al. 2014). This drug candidate is in preclinical development, and, in 2015, it received orphan drug status in the USA for the treatment of chronic inflammatory demyelinating polyradiculoneuropathy (Adis Insight. Research program: autoimmune disorder therapeutics—Gliknik GL-2045. http://adisinsight.springer.com/drugs/800035077).

The knowledge of how IgM polymerizes via Fc domains was leveraged to develop a novel approach to generating recombinant polymeric Fc-fusion proteins. Specifically, more controlled oligomers—hexameric Fc proteins—were generated by Richard Pleass as potential alternatives to IVIg (Czajkowsky et al. 2015; Mekhaiel et al. 2011). These hexameric proteins were shown to bind low-affinity inhibitory receptors FcRL5, FcγRIIb, and DC-SIGN with high avidity and specificity, although they can also activate complement pathways (Czajkowsky et al. 2015). These proteins have yet to advance to the clinic, but they have great potential as more effective and less expensive to produce than IVIg. Another hexameric Fc-fusion protein was created by UCB, which was shown to alter receptor density and trigger internalization and degradation of FcγRs in vitro (Qureshi et al. 2017). As a result, the molecule caused Fc binding disruption and phagocytosis in vitro and the inhibition of platelet phagocytosis in a mouse ITP model. However, the molecule also exhibited a short half-life in mice and cynomolgus monkeys. This work pointed to yet another mechanism through which oligomeric Fc compounds can exert anti-inflammatory activity. This molecule has not been advanced to clinical use. Most recently, CSL generated an rFc hexamer, termed Fc-mTP-L309C, by fusing IgM μ-tailpiece to the C terminus human IgG1-Fc (Spirig et al. 2018). The hexamer bound FcγRs with high avidity and could inhibit a range of in vitro FcγR-mediated effector functions such as ADCC, phagocytosis, and respiratory burst. In addition, the molecule potently inhibited the activation of the classic complement pathway. In vivo, Fc-mTP-L309C suppressed inflammatory arthritis in mice at a 10-fold lower dose than IVIg, and, in a mouse model of immune thrombocytopenia, it successfully restored platelet counts. The authors hypothesize that the mechanism of action exerted by this hexamer is through blockade of FcγRs and through its unique inhibition of complement activation.

The concept of selectively antagonizing the activating FcγR system without activating proinflammatory pathways was introduced by Momenta Pharmaceuticals (Ortiz et al. 2016). Through novel insight into the modulation of the FcγR pathways, a trivalent-IgG-Fc recombinant product candidate—Fc3Y, or M230—was designed. M230 was designed to preferentially assemble into a homogeneous trimeric IgG-Fc using knobs into hole and electrostatic steering molecular heterodimerization technology. Trivalent M230 exerts avid binding to FcγRs, without inadvertently activating immune cell effector functions, resulting in a potent molecule that inhibits immune complex-driven processes in many cells that express FcγRs. A main driver for the design of M230 was the identification of a threshold for activation of the FcγR signaling pathways with Fc-multimers containing five or

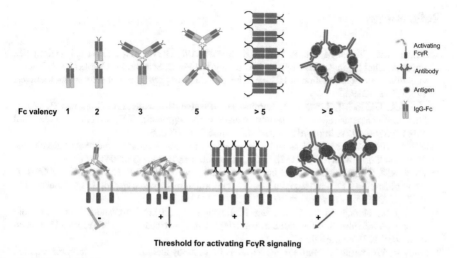

Fig. 3 Schematic representation of the IgG1-Fc valency threshold required for FcγR signaling identified by Bosques and coworkers

more Fc units but not with multivalent Fc containing three or less Fc units (Fig. 3). Furthermore, M230 has been shown to have 40-fold greater potency than IVIg in animal models of autoimmune diseases such as arthritis, immune thrombocytopenia, and epidermolysis bullosa acquisita skin blistering. This drug candidate is in clinical development in collaboration with CSL, and it may represent an effective therapeutic candidate for FcγR-mediated autoimmune diseases.

8 Conclusion

Studies from the past 15 years have shed new light on the mechanisms by which IgG can perform pro- and anti-inflammatory activities. Through detailed biophysical characterization, use of in vitro and in vivo models, and biomarker studies in clinical investigation, the role of glycosylation in the anti-inflammatory and immunoregulatory properties of IgG has been well established. At the molecular level, studies have shown the far-reaching effects of terminal Fc sialylation and have demonstrated the ability of this sugar moiety to modulate Fc structure and interactions with FcRs. In addition to the use of IVIg in the clinic, the relationship between Fc glycosylation states and disease activity in various autoimmune disorders has provided valuable human evidence of the immunoregulatory effects of IgG. Detailed in vitro and in vivo studies have elucidated the key receptors, cells, and signaling cascades involved in these anti-inflammatory processes. This knowledge has enabled the evaluation of new therapeutics, such as multivalent Fc drug candidates and hypersialylated IVIg, which are being developed to harness the anti-inflammatory effects of IgG.

References

Ackerman ME, Crispin M, Yu X, Baruah K, Boesch AW, Harvey DJ, Dugast AS, Heizen EL, Ercan A, Choi I, Streeck H, Nigrovic PA, Bailey-Kelogg C, Scanlan C, Alter G (2013) Natural variation in Fc glycosylation of HIV-specific antibodies impacts antiviral activity. J Clin Invest 123(5):2183–2192

Ahmed AA, Giddens J, Pincetic A, Lomino JV, Ravetch JV, Wang LX, Bjorkman PJ (2014) Structural characterization of anti-inflammatory immunoglobulin G Fc proteins. J Molec Biol 426(18):3166–3179. https://doi.org/10.1016/j.jmb.2014.07.006

Akilesh S (2004) The MHC class I-like Fc receptor promotes humorally mediated autoimmune disease. J Clin Invest 113(9):1328–1333. https://doi.org/10.1172/jci200418838

Anthony RM, Nimmerjahn F, Ashline D, Reinhold V, Paulson J, Ravetch JV (2008a) A recombinant IgG Fc that recapitulates the anti-inflammatory activity of IVIg. Science 320 (5874):373–376. https://doi.org/10.1126/science.1154315

Anthony RM, Kobayashi T, Wermeling F, Ravetch JV (2011) Intravenous gammaglobulin suppresses inflammation through a novel T(H)2 pathway. Nature 475(7354):110–113. https://doi.org/10.1038/nature10134

Anthony R, Wermeling F, Karlsson M, Ravetch JV (2008b) Identification of a receptor required for the anti-inflammatory activity of IVIG. Proc Natl Acad Sci U S A 105(50):19571–19578. https://doi.org/10.1073/pnas.0810163105

Arnold JN, Wormald MR, Sim RB, Rudd PM, Dwek RA (2007) The impact of glycosylation on the biological function and structure of human immunoglobulins. Ann Rev Immunol 25:21–50. https://doi.org/10.1146/annurev.immunol.25.022106.141702

Barreto M, Ferreira RC, Lourenco L, Moraes-Fontes MF, Santos E, Alves M, Carvalho C, Martins B, Andreia R, Viana JF, Vasconcelos C, Mota-Vieira L, Ferreira C, Demengeot J, Vicente AM (2009) Low frequency of CD4$^+$ CD25$^+$ Treg in SLE patients: a heritable trait associated with CTLA4 and TGFβ gene variants. BMC Immunol 10:5. https://doi.org/10.1186/1471-2172-10-5

Bayry J, Lacroix-Desmazes S, Carbonneil C, Misra N, Donkova V, Pashov A, Chevailler A, Mouthon L, Weill B, Bruneval P, Kazatchkine MD, Kaveri SV (2003) Inhibition of maturation and function of dendritic cells by intravenous immunoglobulin. Blood 101(2):758–765. https://doi.org/10.1182/blood-2002-05-1447

Boruchov AM, Heller G, Veri MC, Bonvini E, Ravetch JV, Young JW (2005) Activating and inhibitory IgG Fc receptors on human DCs mediate opposing functions. J Clin Invest 115 (10):2914–2923. https://doi.org/10.1172/JCI24772

Bruhns P, Samuelsson A, Pollard J, Ravetch JV (2003) Colony-stimulating factor-1-dependent macrophages are responsible for IVIG Protection in antibody-induced autoimmune disease. Immunity 18(4):573–581. https://doi.org/10.1016/S1074-7613(03)00080-3

Bruhns P, Iannascoli B, England P, Mancardi D, Fernandez N, Jorieux S, Daeron M (2009) Specificity and affinity of human Fcγ receptors and their polymorphic variants for human IgG subclasses. Blood 113(16):3716–3725. https://doi.org/10.1182/blood2008-09-179754

Burns JC, Franco A (2015) The immunomodulatory effects of intravenous immunoglobulin therapy in Kawasaki disease. Expert Rev Clin Immunol 11(7):819–825. https://doi.org/10.1586/1744666X.2015.1044980

Burns JC, Song Y, Bujold M, Shimizu C, Kanegaye JT, Tremoulet AH, Franco A (2013) Immune-monitoring in Kawasaki disease patients treated with infliximab and intravenous immunoglobulin. Clin Exp Immunol 174(3):337–344. https://doi.org/10.1111/cei.12182

Burton OT, Logsdon SL, Zhou JS, Medina-Tamayo J, Abdel-Gadir A, Noval Rivas M, Koleoglou KJ, Chatila TA, Schneider LC, Rachid R, Umetsu DT, Oettgen HC (2014) Oral immunotherapy induces IgG antibodies that act through FcγRIIb to suppress IgE-mediated hypersensitivity. J Allergy Clin Immunol 134(6):1310–1317 e1316. https://doi.org/10.1016/j.jaci.2014.05.042

Chi LJ, Wang HB, Zhang Y, Wang WZ (2007) Abnormality of circulating CD4(+) CD25(+) regulatory T cell in patients with Guillain-Barre syndrome. J Neuroimmunol 192(1–2):206–214. https://doi.org/10.1016/j.jneuroim.2007.09.034

Chu SY, Vostiar I, Karki S, Moore GL, Lazar GA, Pong E, Joyce PF, Szymkowski DE, Desjarlais JR (2008) Inhibition of B cell receptor-mediated activation of primary human B cells by coengagement of CD19 and FcγRIIb with Fc-engineered antibodies. Mol Immunol 45 (15):3926–3933. https://doi.org/10.1016/j.molimm.2008.06.027

Cines DB, Bussel JB (2005) How I treat idiopathic thrombocytopenic purpura (ITP). Blood 106 (7):2244–2251. https://doi.org/10.1182/blood-2004-12-4598

Clynes RA, Towers TL, Presta LG, Ravetch JV (2000) Inhibitory Fc receptors modulate in vivo cytoxicity against tumor targets. Nat Med 6(4):443–446

Crow AR, Song S, Freedman J, Helgason CD, Humphries RK, Siminovitch KA, Lazarus AH (2003) IVIg-mediated amelioration of murine ITP via FcγRIIB is independent of SHIP1, SHP-1, and Btk activity. Blood 102(2):558–560. https://doi.org/10.1182/blood-2003-01-0023

Czajkowsky DM, Andersen JT, Fuchs A, Wilson TJ, Mekhaiel D, Colonna M, He J, Shao Z, Mitchell DA, Wu G, Dell A, Haslam S, Lloyd KA, Moore SC, Sandlie I, Blundell PA, Pleass RJ (2015) Developing the IVIG biomimetic, hexa-Fc, for drug and vaccine applications. Sci Rep 5:9526. https://doi.org/10.1038/srep09526

De Groot AS, Moise L, McMurry JA, Wambre E, Van Overtvelt L, Moingeon P, Scott DW, Martin W (2008) Activation of natural regulatory T cells by IgG Fc-derived peptide "Tregitopes". Blood 112(8):3303–3311. https://doi.org/10.1182/blood-2008-02-138073

Debre M, Griscelli C, Bonnet MC, Carosella E, Philippe N, Reinert P, Vilmer E, Kaplan C, Fridman WH, Teillaud JL (1993) Infusion of Fcγ fragments for treatment of children with acute immune thrombocytopenic purpura. Lancet 342(8877):945–949. https://doi.org/10.1016/0140-6736(93)92000-J

Delfraissy JF, Tchernia G, Laurian Y, Wallon C, Galanaud P, Dormont J (1985) Suppressor cell function after intravenous gammaglobulin treatment in adult chronic idiopathic thrombocytopenic purpura. Br J Haematol 60(2):315–322. https://doi.org/10.1111/j.1365-2141.1985.tb07417.x

Dube R, Rook GA, Steele J, Brealey R, Dwek RA, Rademacher T, Lennard-Jones J (1990) Agalactosyl IgG in inflammatory bowel disease: correlation with C-reactive protein. Gut 31 (4):431–434. https://doi.org/10.1136/gut.31.4.431

Durandy A, Fischer A, Griscelli C (1981) Dysfunctions of pokeweed mitogen-stimulated T and B lymphocyte responses induced by gammaglobulin therapy. J Clin Invest 67(3):867–877. https://doi.org/10.1172/JCI110104

Engdahl C, Bondt A, Harre U, Raufer J, Pfeifle R, Camponeschi A, Wuhrer M, Seeling M, Martensson IL, Nimmerjahn F, Kronke G, Scherer HU, Forsblad-d'Elia H, Schett G (2018) Estrogen induces St6gal1 expression and increases IgG sialylation in mice and patients with rheumatoid arthritis: a potential explanation for the increased risk of rheumatoid arthritis in postmenopausal women. Arthritis Res Ther 20(1):84. https://doi.org/10.1186/s13075-018-1586-z

Ephrem A, Chamat S, Miquel C, Fisson S, Mouthon L, Caligiuri G, Delignat S, Elluru S, Bayry J, Lacroix-Desmazes S, Cohen JL, Salomon BL, Kazatchkine MD, Kaveri SV, Misra N (2008) Expansion of CD4$^+$ CD25$^+$ regulatory T cells by intravenous immunoglobulin: a critical factor in controlling experimental autoimmune encephalomyelitis. Blood 111(2):715–722. https://doi.org/10.1182/blood-2007-03-079947

Epp A, Hobusch J, Bartsch YC, Petry J, Lilienthal GM, Koeleman CAM, Eschweiler S, Mobs C, Hall A, Morris SC, Braumann D, Engellenner C, Bitterling J, Rahmoller J, Leliavski A, Thurmann R, Collin M, Moremen KW, Strait RT, Blanchard V, Petersen A, Gemoll T, Habermann JK, Petersen F, Nandy A, Kahlert H, Hertl M, Wuhrer M, Pfutzner W, Jappe U, Finkelman FD, Ehlers M (2018) Sialylation of IgG antibodies inhibits IgG-mediated allergic reactions. J Allergy Clin Immunol 141(1):399–402 e398. https://doi.org/10.1016/j.jaci.2017.06.021

Espy C, Morelle W, Kavian N, Grange P, Goulvestre C, Viallon V, Chereau C, Pagnoux C, Michalski JC, Guillevin L, Weill B, Batteux F, Guilpain P (2011) Sialylation levels of anti-proteinase 3 antibodies are associated with the activity of granulomatosis with polyangiitis (Wegener's). Arthritis Rheum 63(7):2105–2115. https://doi.org/10.1002/art.30362

Feige MJ, Nath S, Catharino SR, Weinfurtner D, Steinbacher S, Buchner J (2009) Structure of the murine unglycosylated IgG1 Fc fragment. J Molec Biol 391(3):599–608. https://doi.org/10.1016/j.jmb.2009.06.048

Ferrara C, Grau S, Jager C, Sondermann P, Brunker P, Waldhauer I, Hennig M, Ruf A, Rufer AC, Stihle M, Umana P, Benz J (2011) Unique carbohydrate–carbohydrate interactions are required for high affinity binding between FcγRIII and antibodies lacking core fucose. Proc Natl Acad Sci U S A 108(31):12669–12674. https://doi.org/10.1073/pnas.1108455108

Fickentscher C, Magorivska I, Janko C, Biermann M, Bilyy R, Nalli C, Tincani A, Medeghini V, Meini A, Nimmerjahn F, Schett G, Munoz LE, Andreoli L, Herrmann M (2015) The Pathogenicity of anti-β2GP1-IgG Autoantibodies depends on Fc glycosylation. J Immunol Res 2015:638129. https://doi.org/10.1155/2015/638129

Fiebiger BM, Maamary J, Pincetic A, Ravetch JV (2015) Protection in antibody- and T cell-mediated autoimmune diseases by antiinflammatory IgG Fcs requires type II FcRs. Proc Natl Acad Sci U S A 112(18):E2385–E2394. https://doi.org/10.1073/pnas.1505292112

Fokkink WJ, Selman MH, Dortland JR, Durmus B, Kuitwaard K, Huizinga R, van Rijs W, Tio-Gillen AP, van Doorn PA, Deelder AM, Wuhrer M, Jacobs BC (2014) IgG Fc N-glycosylation in Guillain-Barre syndrome treated with immunoglobulins. J Proteome Res 13 (3):1722–1730. https://doi.org/10.1021/pr401213z

Franco A, Touma R, Song Y, Shimizu C, Tremoulet AH, Kanegaye JT, Burns JC (2014) Specificity of regulatory T cells that modulate vascular inflammation. Autoimmunity 47(2):95–104. https://doi.org/10.3109/08916934.2013.860524

Gringhuis SI, Kaptein TM, Wevers BA, van der Vlist M, Klaver EJ, van Die I, Vriend LE, de Jong MA, Geijtenbeek TB (2014) Fucose-based PAMPs prime dendritic cells for follicular T helper cell polarization via DC-SIGN-dependent IL-27 production. Nat Commun 5:5074. https://doi.org/10.1038/ncomms6074

Gupta A, Novik BE, Rubinstein A (1986) Restoration of suppressor T-cell functions in children With AIDS following intravenous gamma globulin treatment. Am J Dis Child 140(2):143–146. https://doi.org/10.1001/archpedi.1986.02140160061033

Hansen RJ, Balthasar JP (2002) Effects of intravenous immunoglobulin on platelet count and antiplatelet antibodydisposition in a rat model of immune thrombocytopenia. Blood 100 (6):2087–2093

Harre U, Lang SC, Pfeifle R, Rombouts Y, Fruhbeisser S, Amara K, Bang H, Lux A, Koeleman CA, Baum W, Dietel K, Grohn F, Malmstrom V, Klareskog L, Kronke G, Kocijan R, Nimmerjahn F, Toes RE, Herrmann M, Scherer HU, Schett G (2015) Glycosylation of immunoglobulin G determines osteoclast differentiation and bone loss. Nat Commun 6:6651. https://doi.org/10.1038/ncomms7651

Heyman B (2003) Feedback regulation by IgG antibodies. Immunol Lett 88(2):157–161. https://doi.org/10.1016/s0165-2478(03)00078-6

Houde D, Peng Y, Berkowitz S, Engen JR (2010) Post-translational modifications differentially affect IgG1 conformation and receptor binding. Mol Cell Proteomics 9(8):1716–1728. https://doi.org/10.1074/mcp.M900540-MCP200

Huang HS, Sun DS, Lien TS, Chang HH (2010) Dendritic cells modulate platelet activity in IVIg-mediated amelioration of ITP in mice. Blood 116(23):5002–5009. https://doi.org/10.1182/blood-2010-03-275123

Jain A, Olsen HS, Vyzasatya R, Burch E, Sakoda Y, Merigeon EY, Cai L, Lu C, Tan M, Tamada K, Schulze D, Block DS, Strome SE (2012) Fully recombinant IgG2a Fc multimers (stradomers) effectively treat collagen-induced arthritis and prevent idiopathic thrombocytopenic purpura in mice. Arthritis Res Ther 14(4):R192

Jefferis R, Lund J (2002) Interaction sites on human IgG-Fc for FcγR: current models. Immunol Lett 82(1–2):57–65

Kanazawa N (2007) Dendritic cell immunoreceptors: C-type lectin receptors for pattern-recognition and signaling on antigen-presenting cells. J Dermatol Sci 45(2):77–86. https://doi.org/10.1016/j.jdermsci.2006.09.001

Kaneko Y, Nimmerjahn F, Madaio MP, Ravetch JV (2006a) Pathology and protection in nephrotoxic nephritis is determined by selective engagement of specific Fc receptors. J Exp Med 203(3):789–797. https://doi.org/10.1084/jem.20051900

Kaneko Y, Nimmerjahn F, Ravetch JV (2006b) Anti-inflammatory activity of immunoglobulin G resulting from Fc sialylation. Science 313(5787):670–673. https://doi.org/10.1126/science.1129594

Kao D, Lux A, Schaffert A, Lang R, Altmann F, Nimmerjahn F (2017) IgG subclass and vaccination stimulus determine changes in antigen specific antibody glycosylation in mice. Eur J Immunol 47(12):2070–2079. https://doi.org/10.1002/eji.201747208

Kapur R, Della Valle L, Sonneveld M, Hipgrave Ederveen A, Visser R, Ligthart P, de Haas M, Wuhrer M, van der Schoot CE, Vidarsson G (2014a) Low anti-RhD IgG-Fc-fucosylation in pregnancy: a new variable predicting severity in haemolytic disease of the fetus and newborn. Br J Haematol 166(6):936–945. https://doi.org/10.1111/bjh.12965

Kapur R, Kustiawan I, Vestrheim A, Koeleman CA, Visser R, Einarsdottir HK, Porcelijn L, Jackson D, Kumpel B, Deelder AM, Blank D, Skogen B, Killie MK, Michaelsen TE, de Haas M, Rispens T, van der Schoot CE, Wuhrer M, Vidarsson G (2014b) A prominent lack of IgG1-Fc fucosylation of platelet alloantibodies in pregnancy. Blood 123(4):471–480. https://doi.org/10.1182/blood-2013-09-527978

Kaufman GN, Massoud AH, Audusseau S, Banville-Langelier AA, Wang Y, Guay J, Garellek JA, Mourad W, Piccirillo CA, McCusker C, Mazer BD (2011) Intravenous immunoglobulin attenuates airway hyperresponsiveness in a murine model of allergic asthma. Clin Exp Allergry 41(5):718–728. https://doi.org/10.1111/j.1365-2222.2010.03663.x

Kemna MJ, Plomp R, van Paassen P, Koeleman CAM, Jansen BC, Damoiseaux J, Cohen Tervaert JW, Wuhrer M (2017) Galactosylation and sialylation levels of IgG predict relapse in patients with PR3-ANCA associated vasculitis. EBioMedicine 17:108–118. https://doi.org/10.1016/j.ebiom.2017.01.033

Kiener PA, Lioubin MN, Rohrschneider LR, Ledbetter JA, Nadler SG, Diegel ML (1997) Co-ligation of the antigen and Fc receptors gives rise to the selective modulation of intracellular signaling in B cells. J Biol Chem 272(6):3838–3844

Krapp S, Mimura Y, Jefferis R, Huber R, Sondermann P (2003) Structural analysis of human IgG-Fc glycoforms reveals a correlation between glycosylation and structural integrity. J Mol Biol 325(5):979–989. https://doi.org/10.1016/s0022-2836(02)01250-0

Kurowska W, Kuca-Warnawin EH, Radzikowska A, Maslinski W (2017) The role of anti-citrullinated protein antibodies (ACPA) in the pathogenesis of rheumatoid arthritis. Cent Eur J Immunol 42(4):390–398. https://doi.org/10.5114/ceji.2017.72807

Leontyev D, Katsman Y, Ma XZ, Miescher S, Kasermann F, Branch DR (2012) Sialylation-independent mechanism involved in the amelioration of murine immune thrombocytopenia using intravenous gammaglobulin. Transfusion 52(8):1799–1805. https://doi.org/10.1111/j.1537-2995.2011.03517.x

Li N, Zhao M, Hilario-Vargas J, Prisayanh P, Warren S, Diaz LA, Roopenian DC, Liu Z (2005) Complete FcRn dependence for intravenous Ig therapy in autoimmune skin blistering diseases. J Clin Invest 115(12):3440–3450. https://doi.org/10.1172/JCI24394

Li T, DiLillo DJ, Bournazos S, Giddens JP, Ravetch JV, Wang LX (2017) Modulating IgG effector function by Fc glycan engineering. Proc Natl Acad Sci U S A 114(13):3485–3490. https://doi.org/10.1073/pnas.1702173114

Lood C, Allhorn M, Lood R, Gullstrand B, Olin AI, Ronnblom L, Truedsson L, Collin M, Bengtsson AA (2012) IgG glycan hydrolysis by endoglycosidase S diminishes the proinflammatory properties of immune complexes from patients with systemic lupus erythematosus: a possible new treatment? Arthritis Rheum 64(8):2698–2706. https://doi.org/10.1002/art.34454

Maamary J, Wang TT, Tan GS, Palese P, Ravetch JV (2017) Increasing the breadth and potency of response to the seasonal influenza virus vaccine by immune complex immunization. Proc Natl Acad Sci U S A 114(38):10172–10177

Maddur MS, Stephen-Victor E, Das M, Prakhar P, Sharma VK, Singh V, Rabin M, Trinath J, Balaji KN, Bolgert F, Vallat JM, Magy L, Kaveri SV, Bayry J (2017) Regulatory T cell frequency, but not plasma IL-33 levels, represents potential immunological biomarker to predict clinical response to intravenous immunoglobulin therapy. J Neuroinflammation 14 (1):58. https://doi.org/10.1186/s12974-017-0818-5

Magorivska I, Munoz LE, Janko C, Dumych T, Rech J, Schett G, Nimmerjahn F, Bilyy R, Herrmann M (2016) Sialylation of anti-histone immunoglobulin G autoantibodies determines their capabilities to participate in the clearance of late apoptotic cells. Clin Exp Immunol 184 (1):110–117. https://doi.org/10.1111/cei.12744

Massoud AH, Guay J, Shalaby KH, Bjur E, Ablona A, Chan D, Nouhi Y, McCusker CT, Mourad MW, Piccirillo CA, Mazer BD (2012) Intravenous immunoglobulin attenuates airway inflammation through induction of forkhead box protein 3-positive regulatory T cells. J Allergy Clin Immunol 129(6):1656–1665 e1653. https://doi.org/10.1016/j.jaci.2012.02.050

Massoud AH, Yona M, Xue D, Chouiali F, Alturaihi H, Ablona A, Mourad W, Piccirillo CA, Mazer BD (2014) Dendritic cell immunoreceptor: a novel receptor for intravenous immunoglobulin mediates induction of regulatory T cells. J Allergy Clin Immunol 133 (3):853–863 e855. https://doi.org/10.1016/j.jaci.2013.09.029

Mekhaiel DN, Czajkowsky DM, Andersen JT, Shi J, El-Faham M, Doenhoff M, McIntosh RS, Sandlie I, He J, Hu J, Shao Z, Pleass RJ (2011) Polymeric human Fc-fusion proteins with modified effector functions. Sci Rep 1:124. https://doi.org/10.1038/srep00124

Mimura Y, Church S, Ghirlando R, Ashton PR, Dong S, Goodall M, Lund J, Jefferis R (2000) The influence of glycosylation on the thermal stability and effector function expression of human IgG1-Fc: properties of a series of truncated glycoforms. Mol Immunol 37(12):697–706

Mimura Y, Sondermann P, Ghirlando R, Lund J, Young SP, Goodall M, Jefferis R (2001) Role of oligosaccharide residues of IgG1-Fc in FcγRIIb binding. J Biol Chem 276(49):45539–45547. https://doi.org/10.1074/jbc.M107478200

Mogensen TH, Melchjorsen J, Larsen CS, Paludan SR (2010) Innate immune recognition and activation during HIV infection. Retrovirology 7:54. https://doi.org/10.1186/1742-4690-7-54

Nechansky A, Schuster M, Jost W, Siegl P, Wiederkum S, Gorr G, Kircheis R (2007) Compensation of endogenous IgG mediated inhibition of antibody-dependent cellular cytotoxicity by glyco-engineering of therapeutic antibodies. Mol Immunol 44(7):1815–1817. https://doi.org/10.1016/j.molimm.2006.08.013

Niknami M, Wang MX, Nguyen T, Pollard JD (2013) Beneficial effect of a multimerized immunoglobulin Fc in an animal model of inflammatory neuropathy (experimental autoimmune neuritis). J Peripher Nerv Syst 18(2):141–152

Nimmerjahn F, Ravetch JV (2005) Divergent immunoglobulin G subclass activity through selective Fc receptor binding. Science 310(5759):1510–1512

Nimmerjahn F, Ravetch JV (2006) Fcγ receptors: old friends and new family members. Immunity 24(1):19–28. https://doi.org/10.1016/j.immuni.2005.11.010

Nose M, Wigzell H (1983) Biological significance of carbohydrate chains on monoclonal antibodies. Proc Natl Acad Sci U S A 80(21):6632–6636

Oefner CM, Winkler A, Hess C, Lorenz AK, Holecska V, Huxdorf M, Schommartz T, Petzold D, Bitterling J, Schoen AL, Stoehr AD, Vu Van D, Darcan-Nikolaisen Y, Blanchard V, Schmudde I, Laumonnier Y, Strover HA, Hegazy AN, Eiglmeier S, Schoen CT, Mertes MM, Loddenkemper C, Lohning M, Konig P, Petersen A, Luger EO, Collin M, Kohl J, Hutloff A, Hamelmann E, Berger M, Wardemann H, Ehlers M (2012) Tolerance induction with T cell-dependent protein antigens induces regulatory sialylated IgGs. J Allergy Clin Immunol 129(6):1647–1655 e1613. https://doi.org/10.1016/j.jaci.2012.02.037

Ogata S, Shimizu C, Franco A, Touma R, Kanegaye JT, Choudhury BP, Naidu NN, Kanda Y, Hoang LT, Hibberd ML, Tremoulet AH, Varki A, Burns JC (2013) Treatment response in Kawasaki disease is associated with sialylation levels of endogenous but not therapeutic intravenous immunoglobulin. G. PLoS ONE 8(12):e81448. https://doi.org/10.1371/journal. pone.0081448

Ohkuma K, Sasaki T, Kamei S, Okuda S, Nakano H, Hamamoto T, Fujihara K, Nakashima I, Misu T, Itoyama Y (2007) Modulation of dendritic cell development by immunoglobulin G in control subjects and multiple sclerosis patients. Clin Exp Immunol 150(3):397–406. https://doi. org/10.1111/j.1365-2249.2007.03496.x

Ohmi Y, Ise W, Harazono A, Takakura D, Fukuyama H, Baba Y, Narazaki M, Shoda H, Takahashi N, Ohkawa Y, Ji S, Sugiyama F, Fujio K, Kumanogoh A, Yamamoto K, Kawasaki N, Kurosaki T, Takahashi Y, Furukawa K (2016) Sialylation converts arthritogenic IgG into inhibitors of collagen-induced arthritis. Nat Commun 7:11205. https://doi.org/10. 1038/ncomms11205

Ono M, Okada H, Bolland S, Yanagi S, Tomohiro K, Ravetch JV (1997) Deletion of SHIP or SHP-1 reveals two distinct pathways for inhibitory signaling. Cell 90(2):293–301

Ortiz DF, Lansing JC, Rutitzky L, E. K, Prod'homme T, Choudhury A, Washburn N, Bhatnagar N, Beneduce C, K. H, Prenovitz R, Child M, Killough J, Tyler S, Brown J, Nguyen S, Schwab I, Hains M, Meccariello R, Markowitz L, Wang J, Zouaoui R, Simpson A, Schultes B, Capila I, Ling L, Nimmerjahn F, Manning AM, Bosques CJ (2016) Elucidating the interplay between IgG-Fc valency and FcγR activation for the design of immune complex inhibitors. Sci Transl Med 8(365):ra158

Pagan JD, Kitaoka M, Anthony RM (2018) Engineered sialylation of pathogenic antibodies in vivo attenuates autoimmune disease. Cell 172(3):564–577 e513. https://doi.org/10.1016/j. cell.2017.11.041

Parekh RB, Dwek RA, Sutton BJ, Fernandes DL, Leung A, Stanworth D, Rademacher T, Mizouchi T, Takahashi N, Matsuta K (1985) Association of rheumatoid arthritis and primary osteoarthritis with changes in the glycosylation pattern of total serum IgG. Nature 316

Pasek M, Duk M, Podbielska M, Sokolik R, Szechinski J, Lisowska E, Krotkiewski H (2006) Galactosylation of IgG from rheumatoid arthritis (RA) patients—changes during therapy. Glycoconjugate J 23(7–8):463–471. https://doi.org/10.1007/s10719-006-5409-0

Qian J, Zhu J, Wang M, Wu S, Chen T (2011) Suppressive effects of intravenous immunoglobulin (IVIG) on human umbilical cord blood immune cells. Pediatr Allergy Immunol 22(2):211–220. https://doi.org/10.1111/j.1399-3038.2010.01049.x

Qureshi OS, Rowley TF, Junker F, Peters SJ, Crilly S, Compson J, Eddleston A, Bjorkelund H, Greenslade K, Parkinson M, Davies NL, Griffin R, Pither TL, Cain K, Christodoulou L, Staelens L, Ward E, Tibbitts J, Kiessling A, Smith B, Brennan FR, Malmqvist M, Fallah-Arani F, Humphreys DP (2017) Multivalent Fcγ-receptor engagement by a hexameric Fc-fusion protein triggers Fcγ-receptor internalisation and modulation of Fcγ-receptor functions. Sci Rep 7(1):17049. https://doi.org/10.1038/s41598-017-17255-8

Raju TS (2008) Terminal sugars of Fc glycans influence antibody effector functions of IgGs. Curr Opin Immunol 20(4):471–478. https://doi.org/10.1016/j.coi.2008.06.007

Ramakrishna C, Newo AN, Shen YW, Cantin E (2011) Passively administered pooled human immunoglobulins exert IL-10 dependent anti-inflammatory effects that protect against fatal HSV encephalitis. PLoS Pathog 7(6):e1002071. https://doi.org/10.1371/journal.ppat.1002071

Ravetch JV, Clynes RA (1998) Divergent roles for Fc receptors and complement in vivo. Ann Rev Immunol 16:421–432

Rombouts Y, Ewing E, van de Stadt LA, Selman MH, Trouw LA, Deelder AM, Huizinga TW, Wuhrer M, van Schaardenburg D, Toes RE, Scherer HU (2015) Anti-citrullinated protein antibodies acquire a pro-inflammatory Fc glycosylation phenotype prior to the onset of rheumatoid arthritis. Ann Rheum Dis 74(1):234–241. https://doi.org/10.1136/annrheumdis-2013-203565

Rook GA, Steele J, Brealey R, Whyte A, Isenberg D, Sumar N, Nelson JL, Bodman KB, Young A, Roitt IM (1991) Changes in IgG glycoform levels are associated with remission of arthritis during pregnancy. J Autoimmun 4(5):779–794

Samuelsson A, Towers TL, Ravetch JV (2001) Anti-inflammatory activity of IVIG mediated through the inhibitory Fc receptor. Science 291(5503):484–486

Scallon BJ, Tam SH, McCarthy SG, Cai AN, Raju TS (2007) Higher levels of sialylated Fc glycans in immunoglobulin G molecules can adversely impact functionality. Mol Immunol 44 (7):1524–1534. https://doi.org/10.1016/j.molimm.2006.09.005

Scherer HU, van der Woude D, Ioan-Facsinay A, el Bannoudi H, Trouw LA, Wang J, Haupl T, Burmester GR, Deelder AM, Huizinga TW, Wuhrer M, Toes RE (2010) Glycan profiling of anti-citrullinated protein antibodies isolated from human serum and synovial fluid. Arthritis Rheum 62(6):1620–1629. https://doi.org/10.1002/art.27414

Schwab I, Nimmerjahn F (2013) Intravenous immunoglobulin therapy: how does IgG modulate the immune system? Nat Rev Immunol 13(3):176–189. https://doi.org/10.1038/nri3401

Schwab I, Biburger M, Kronke G, Schett G, Nimmerjahn F (2012) IVIg-mediated amelioration of ITP in mice is dependent on sialic acid and SIGNR1. Eur J Immunol 42(4):826–830. https://doi.org/10.1002/eji.201142260

Schwab I, Mihai S, Seeling M, Kasperkiewicz M, Ludwig RJ, Nimmerjahn F (2014) Broad requirement for terminal sialic acid residues and FcγRIIB for the preventive and therapeutic activity of intravenous immunoglobulins in vivo. Eur J Immunol 44(5):1444–1453. https://doi.org/10.1002/eji.201344230

Selman MH, Niks EH, Titulaer MJ, Verschuuren JJ, Wuhrer M, Deelder AM (2011) IgG fc N-glycosylation changes in Lambert-Eaton myasthenic syndrome and myasthenia gravis. J Proteome Res 10(1):143–152

Shields RL, Lai J, Keck R, O'Connell LY, Hong K, Meng YG, Weikert SH, Presta LG (2002) Lack of fucose on human IgG1N-linked oligosaccharide improves binding to human FcγRIII and antibody-dependent cellular toxicity. J Biol Chem 277(30):26733–26740. https://doi.org/10.1074/jbc.M202069200

Shinkawa T, Nakamura K, Yamane N, Shoji-Hosaka E, Kanda Y, Sakurada M, Uchida K, Anazawa H, Satoh M, Yamasaki M, Hanai N, Shitara K (2003) The absence of fucose but not the presence of galactose or bisecting N-acetylglucosamine of human IgG1 complex-type oligosaccharides shows the critical role of enhancing antibody-dependent cellular cytotoxicity. J Biol Chem 278(5):3466–3473. https://doi.org/10.1074/jbc.M210665200

Siragam V, Brinc D, Crow AR, Song S, Freedman J, Lazarus AH (2005) Can antibodies with specificity for soluble antigens mimic the therapeutic effects of intravenous IgG in the treatment of autoimmune disease. J Clin Invest 115(1):155–160. https://doi.org/10.1172/jci200522753ds1

Siragam V, Crow AR, Brinc D, Song S, Freedman J, Lazarus AH (2006) Intravenous immunoglobulin ameliorates ITP via activating Fcγ receptors on dendritic cells. Nat Med 12 (6):688–692. https://doi.org/10.1038/nm1416

Sjowall C, Zapf J, von Lohneysen S, Magorivska I, Biermann M, Janko C, Winkler S, Bilyy R, Schett G, Herrmann M, Munoz LE (2015) Altered glycosylation of complexed native IgG molecules is associated with disease activity of systemic lupus erythematosus. Lupus 24 (6):569–581

Sondermann P, Kaiser J, Jacob U (2001) Molecular basis for immune complex recognition: a comparison of Fc-receptor structures. J Mol Biol 309(3):737–749

Sondermann P, Pincetic A, Maamary J, Lammens K, Ravetch JV (2013) General mechanism for modulating immunoglobulin effector function. Proc Natl Acad Sci U S A 110(24):9868–9872

Sonneveld ME, Natunen S, Sainio S, Koeleman CA, Holst S, Dekkers G, Koelewijn J, Partanen J, van der Schoot CE, Wuhrer M, Vidarsson G (2016) Glycosylation pattern of anti-platelet IgG is stable during pregnancy and predicts clinical outcome in alloimmune thrombocytopenia. Br J Haematol 174(2):310–320. https://doi.org/10.1111/bjh.14053

Sonneveld ME, Koelewijn J, de Haas M, Admiraal J, Plomp R, Koeleman CA, Hipgrave Ederveen AL, Ligthart P, Wuhrer M, van der Schoot CE, Vidarsson G (2017) Antigen specificity determines anti-red blood cell IgG-Fc alloantibody glycosylation and thereby severity of haemolytic disease of the fetus and newborn. Br J Haematol 176(4):651–660. https://doi.org/10.1111/bjh.14438

Spirig R, Campbell IK, Koernig S, Chen CG, Lewis BJB, Butcher R, Muir I, Taylor S, Chia J, Leong D, Simmonds J, Scotney P, Schmidt P, Fabri L, Hofmann A, Jordi M, Spycher MO,

Cattepoel S, Brasseit J, Panousis C, Rowe T, Branch DR, Baz Morelli A, Kasermann F, Zuercher AW (2018) rIgG1 Fc Hexamer inhibits antibody-mediated autoimmune disease via effects on complement and FcγRs. J Immunol 200(8):2542–2553. https://doi.org/10.4049/jimmunol.1701171

Steiniger B, Barth P, Herbst B, Hartnell A, Crocker PR (1997) The species-specific structure of microanatomical compartments in the human spleen: strongly sialoadhesin-positive macrophages occur in the perifollicular zone, but not in the marginal zone. Immunology 92(2):307–316

Strait RT, Morris SC, Finkelman FD (2006) IgG-blocking antibodies inhibit IgE-mediated anaphylaxis in vivo through both antigen interception and FcγRIIb cross-linking. J Clin Invest 116(3):833–841. https://doi.org/10.1172/JCI25575

Subedi GP, Barb AW (2016) The immunoglobulin G1 N-glycan composition affects binding to each low affinity Fcγ receptor. mAbs 8(8):1512–1524. https://doi.org/10.1080/19420862.2016.1218586

Tackenberg B, Jelcic I, Baerenwaldt A, Oertel WH, Sommer N, Nimmerjahn F, Lunemann JD (2009) Impaired inhibitory Fcγ receptor IIB expression on B cells in chronic inflammatory demyelinating polyneuropathy. Proc Natl Acad Sci U S A 106(12):4788–4792. https://doi.org/10.1073/pnas.0807319106

Teeling JL, Jansen-Hendriks T, Juijpers TW, de Haas M, van de Winkel JG, Hack CE, Bleeker WK (2001) Therapeutic efficacy of intravenous immunoglobulin preparations depends on the immunoglobulin G dimers: studies in experimental immune thrombocytopenia. Blood 98(4):1095–1099

Thiruppathi M, Sheng JR, Li L, Prabhakar BS, Meriggioli MN (2014) Recombinant IgG2a Fc (M045) multimers effectively suppress experimental autoimmune myasthenia gravis. J Autoimmun 52:64–73. https://doi.org/10.1016/j.jaut.2013.12.014

Tjon AS, van Gent R, Jaadar H, Martin van Hagen P, Mancham S, van der Laan LJ, te Boekhorst PA, Metselaar HJ, Kwekkeboom J (2014) Intravenous immunoglobulin treatment in humans suppresses dendritic cell function via stimulation of IL-4 and IL-13 production. J Immunol 192(12):5625–5634. https://doi.org/10.4049/jimmunol.1301260

Trbojevic Akmacic I, Ventham NT, Theodoratou E, Vuckovic F, Kennedy NA, Kristic J, Nimmo ER, Kalla R, Drummond H, Stambuk J, Dunlop MG, Novokmet M, Aulchenko Y, Gornik O, Campbell H, Pucic Bakovic M, Satsangi J, Lauc G, Consortium I-B (2015) Inflammatory bowel disease associates with proinflammatory potential of the immunoglobulin G glycome. Inflamm Bowel Dis 21(6):1237–1247. https://doi.org/10.1097/MIB.0000000000000372

Tsurikisawa N, Saito H, Oshikata C, Tsuburai T, Akiyama K (2012) High-dose intravenous immunoglobulin treatment increases regulatory T cells in patients with eosinophilic granulomatosis with polyangiitis. J Rheumatol 39(5):1019–1025. https://doi.org/10.3899/jrheum.110981

Tsurikisawa N, Saito H, Oshikata C, Tsuburai T, Akiyama K (2014) High-dose intravenous immunoglobulin therapy for eosinophilic granulomatosis with polyangiitis. Clin Transl Allergy 4(38)

Vaccaro C, Zhou J, Ober RJ, Ward ES (2005) Engineering the Fc region of immunoglobulin G to modulate in vivo antibody levels. Nat Biotechnol 23(10):1283–1288. https://doi.org/10.1038/nbt1143

van de Geijn FE, Wuhrer M, Selman MH, Willemsen SP, de Man YA, Deelder AM, Hazes JM, Dolhain RJ (2009) Immunoglobulin G galactosylation and sialylation are associated with pregnancy-induced improvement of rheumatoid arthritis and the postpartum flare: results from a large prospective cohort study. Arthritis Res Ther 11(6):R193. https://doi.org/10.1186/ar2892

Viard I, Wehrli P, Bullani R, Schneider P, Holler N, Salomon D, Hunziker T, Saurat JH, Tschopp J, French LE (1998) Inhibition of toxic epidermal necrolysis by blockade of CD95 with human intravenous immunoglobulin. Science 282(5388):490–493

Vidarsson G, Dekkers G, Rispens T (2014) IgG subclasses and allotypes: from structure to effector functions. Front Immunol 5:520. https://doi.org/10.3389/fimmu.2014.00520

Vuckovic F, Kristic J, Gudelj I, Teruel M, Keser T, Pezer M, Pucic-Bakovic M, Stambuk J, Trbojevic Akmacic I, Barrios C, Pavic T, Menni C, Wang Y, Zhou Y, Cui L, Song H, Zeng Q, Guo X, Pns-Estel BA, Mckeigue P, Leslie Patrick A, Gornik O, Spector TD, Harjacek M, Alarcon-Riquelme M, Molokhia M, Wang W, Luac G (2015) Association of systemic lupus erythematosus with decreased immunosuppressive potential of the IgG glycome. Arthritis Rheumatol 67(11):2798–3789

Washburn N, Schwab I, Ortiz D, Bhatnagar N, Lansing JC, Medeiros A, Tyler S, Mekala D, Cochran E, Sarvaiya H, Garofalo K, Meccariello R, Meador JW 3rd, Rutitzky L, Schultes BC, Ling L, Avery W, Nimmerjahn F, Manning AM, Kaundinya GV, Bosques CJ (2015) Controlled tetra-Fc sialylation of IVIg results in a drug candidate with consistent enhanced anti-inflammatory activity. Proc Natl Acad Sci U S A 112(11):E1297–E1306. https://doi.org/10.1073/pnas.1422481112

Watson M, Rudd PM, Bland M, Dwek RA, Axford JS (1999) Sugar printing rheumatic diseases: a potential method for disease differentiation using immunoglobulin G oligosaccharides. Arthritis Rheum 42(8):1682–1690

Wong AH, Fukami Y, Sudo M, Kokubun N, Hamada S, Yuki N (2016) Sialylated IgG-Fc: a novel biomarker of chronic inflammatory demyelinating polyneuropathy. J Neurol Neurosurg Psychiatry 87(3):257–259. https://doi.org/10.1136/jnnp2014-309964

Wuhrer M, Porcelijn L, Kapur R, Koeleman CA, Deelder AM, De Haas M, Vidarsson G (2009) Regulated glycosylation patterns of IgG during alloimmune responses against human platelet antigens. J Proteome Res 8(2):450–456

Wuhrer M, Selman MH, McDonnell LA, Kumpfel T, Derfuss T, Khademi M, Olsson T, Hohlfeld R, Meinl E, Krumbholz M (2015a) Pro-inflammatory pattern of IgG1 Fc glycosylation in multiple sclerosis cerebrospinal fluid. J Neuroinflammation 12:235. https://doi.org/10.1186/s12974-015-0450-1

Wuhrer M, Stavenhagen K, Koeleman CA, Selman MH, Harper L, Jacobs BC, Savage CO, Jefferis R, Deelder AM, Morgan M (2015b) Skewed Fc glycosylation profiles of anti-proteinase 3 immunoglobulin G1 autoantibodies from granulomatosis with polyangiitis patients show low levels of bisection, galactosylation, and sialylation. J Proteome Res 14(4):1657–1665. https://doi.org/10.1021/pr500780a

Zhang G, Massaad CA, Gao T, Pillai L, Bogdanova N, Ghauri S, Sheikh KA (2016) Sialylated intravenous immunoglobulin suppress anti-ganglioside antibody mediated nerve injury. Exp Neurol 282:49–55. https://doi.org/10.1016/j.expneurol.2016.05.020

Zuercher AW, Spirig R, Baz Morelli A, Kasermann F (2016) IVIG in autoimmune disease—potential next generation biologics. Autoimmun Rev 15(8):781–785. https://doi.org/10.1016/j.autrev.2016.03.018

IgG Fc Glycosylation in Human Immunity

Taia T. Wang

Contents

Abstract Glycosylation of IgG Fc domains is a central mechanism in the diversification of antibody function. Modifications to the core Fc glycan impact antibody function by shifting the balance of Type I and Type II Fc gamma receptors (FcγR) that will be engaged by immune complexes. This, in turn, modulates the effector cells and functions that can be recruited during immune activation. Critically, humans have evolved to regulate Fc glycan modifications for immune homeostasis. Dysregulation in Fc glycan modifications can lead to loss of immune tolerance, symptomatic autoimmunity, and susceptibility to infectious diseases. Here, we discuss IgG Fc glycosylation and its role in human health and disease.

T. T. Wang (✉)
Department of Medicine, Division of Infectious Diseases, Department of Microbiology
and Immunology, Program in Immunology, Stanford University School of Medicine,
Stanford University, Stanford, CA 94305, USA
e-mail: taiawang@stanford.edu

T. T. Wang
Chan Zuckerberg Biohub, San Francisco, CA, USA

Current Topics in Microbiology and Immunology (2019) 423: 63–76
https://doi.org/10.1007/82_2019_152
© Springer Nature Switzerland AG 2019
Published online: 26 February 2019

1 Introduction

Recent studies have defined the considerable heterogeneity that exists among people in specific IgG Fc glycan modifications that impact antibody activity in vivo (Selman et al. 2012a, b; Wang et al. 2015, 2017; Mahan et al. 2016; Mahan et al. 2015). Intriguingly, individuals produce distinct basal repertoires of Fc glycoforms which are quite stable over periods of weeks to months (Wang et al. 2015). Because Fc glycan modifications directly affect the ability of IgGs to recruit various effector cell populations, this heterogeneity is likely a significant driver of immune diversity across the population.

The ability of IgG antibodies to mediate effector functions arises from their capacity to bridge antigen binding through the Fab domain with the recruitment of effector cells through interactions between the Fc domain and FcγRs. Because the majority of FcγRs have low affinity for monomeric IgGs, Fc-FcγR interactions occur when multivalent IgG-antigen immune complexes are formed, thus enabling avidity-based interactions and conferring specificity to the effector cell response.

The structure of the Fc domains contained in a given immune complex determines which effector cells and FcγRs can be engaged by the complex. Fc structure, in turn, is determined by two variables: the IgG subclass and the composition of a complex biantennary glycan that is present on all IgG heavy chains within the CH2 domain. Four IgG subclasses are found in humans (IgG1-4), with IgG1 and IgG3 having highest affinity for activating Type I FcγRs (FcγRI, FcγRIIa, FcγRIIIa). In contrast, IgG2 has highest affinity of all subclasses for the inhibitory FcγR, FcγRIIb (Fig. 1).

The activity of different IgG subclasses is further tuned by modifications to the Fc glycan which can impart diverse and potent effector functions to IgG1s and likely to the other subclasses, though how Fc glycosylation impacts the activity of IgG2, IgG3 and IgG4 has yet to be described. Overall, the composition of IgG

Heterogeneity in IgG Fc repertoires

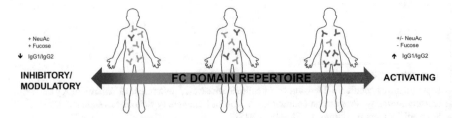

Fig. 1 Heterogeneity in the human IgG Fc domain repertoire. IgG repertoires vary across the population by ratios of activating to inhibitory IgG subclasses ((IgG1+IgG3)/IgG2) and in the abundance of Fc glycoforms that impact Fc domain structure and antibody function. Fucosylated, sialylated Fc glycoforms impart reduced Type I FcγR binding activity and enable binding to the Type II FcγRs. Afucosylated, sialylated or asialylated Fc glycans mediate pro-inflammatory effector functions by virtue of increased affinity for the activating Type I FcγR, FcγRIIIa

subclasses and Fc glycans within immune complexes determines whether they will trigger pro- or anti-inflammatory effector cell activity and regulates the quality of the adaptive immune response against the antigen(s) in complex (Wang et al. 2015; Regnault et al. 1999; Getahun et al. 2004; de Jong et al. 2006; Ding et al. 2016; Hjelm et al. 2008).

2 Structure and Assembly of Fc Glycans

Mature Fc glycoforms are N-linked, complex biantennary structures, present at asparagine 297 of all heavy chains (Kao et al. 2015). The core Fc glycan is composed of seven saccharides and is required for maximal binding to FcγRs: 4 N-acetylglucosamine (GlcNAc) and 3 mannose (Man) residues (Lux et al. 2013). This core glycan can be modified by additional sugars, including a core fucose (Fuc), bisecting GlcNAc, galactose (Gal) at one or both arms and, in the presence of galactose, N-acetylneuraminic acid (NeuAc) or sialic acid (Fig. 2). Two modifications to the IgG1 Fc, fucosylation and sialylation, have well defined functions in vivo and will be discussed in more detail below. How bisecting GlcNAc impacts IgG function is not yet well understood. Some studies indicate a role for bisection in modulation of FcγRIIIa-mediated activities, however data on this are not consistent and any phenotype related to FcgRIIIa binding is clearly less pronounced than what can be achieved through afucosylation of Fc glycans (Hodoniczky et al. 2005; Shinkawa et al. 2003). Galactosylation of the Fc is significant as a precursor to sialylation but does not significantly limit the abundance of Fc sialylation as galactosylation occurs with several fold greater frequency than sialylation (Wang et al. 2015; Wuhrer et al.

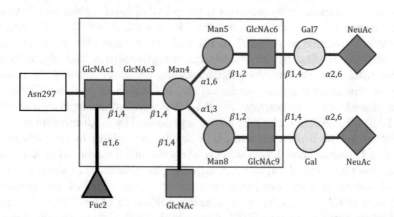

Fig. 2 Structure of IgG Fc glycans. Fc glycoforms are present at Asn 297 within CH2 domains and are complex biantennary glycans. The core Fc glycan (boxed in red) is composed of seven saccharides: 4 N-acetylglucosamine (GlcNAc) and 3 mannose (Man) residues. This core glycan can be modified by a core fucose (Fuc), bisecting GlcNAc, galactose (Gal) at one or both arms and, in the presence of galactose, N-acetyl-neuraminic acid or sialic acid (NeuAc)

Table 1 Set of 11 modifications to the core Fc glycan which, together, comprise ∼90% of human IgG1 Fc glycoforms. Relative quantification of the 11 modifications is shown. G: Galactose; 0,1,2 indicate the number of Gal residues; F: Fucose; N: bisecting GlcNAc; S: sialic acid. Data are from a commercial IVIg preparation

Core glycan modification	IgG1 Fc (% total)
G0	0.18
G1	2.04
G2	3.16
G0F	1.72
G1F	27.11
G2F	38.28
G0FN	0.72
G1FN	7.00
G2FN	0.81
G1FS	1.03
G2FS	17.96
	100.00

2015). A direct role for galactosylated Fc glycans in modulation of immune function has not been defined. Overall, 11 distinct complex biantennary Fc glycoforms comprise ∼90% of the human IgG1 repertoire (Table 1). In addition to complex biantennary glycans, up to ∼2% of Fc glycans on serum IgG1 may be a combination of hybrid and high mannose forms (Flynn et al. 2010 and Wang, unpublished observation).

Assembly of Fc glycans begins with oligomannose forms that are pre-assembled on a lipid, polyprenol dolichol pyrophosphate. The precursor Fc glycan is assembled first by transfer of sugar residues on the cytoplasmic face of the endoplasmic reticulum (ER), followed by transport of the partial precursor across the ER membrane to the luminal side where the full oligomannose N-glycan precursor is assembled. The triantennary precursor is comprised of two GlcNAc, nine Man and three glucose (Glc) residues. Within the ER, this Glc3Man9GlcNac2 oligosaccharide is transferred to Asn 297 of the IgG heavy chain. The Fc glycan then undergoes remodeling by membrane-anchored glycosidases and glycosyltransferases within the ER and the golgi apparatus, ultimately forming the mature, complex, biantennary glycan structure (Fig. 2). Addition of bisecting GlcNAc is accomplished by the activity of β-1,4-*N*-Acetylglucosaminyltransferase III (GNT-III) while addition of a core fucose is performed by α-1,6-fucosyltransferase (FUT8). It has been observed that FUT8 activity is inhibited by the presence of bisecting GlcNAc. Thus, fucosylation is likely the initial modification in glycans that are both fucosylated and bisected. Increasing the abundance of afucosylated Fc glycoforms in in vitro expression systems has been achieved by increasing expression of GNT-III and/or by engineering localization of GNT-III to the upper golgi where it can act prior to FUT8 (Ferrara et al. 2006). Galactosylation of one or both arms of the bisected Fc glycan is performed by β-1,4-galactosyltransferase 1 (B4GALT1) and, in the presence of galactosylation, terminal sialylation is catalyzed by α-2,6-sialyltransferase 1 (ST6GAL1) which preferentially adds sialic acid to the α-1,3 arm of the biantennary glycan (Barb et al. 2009).

3   IgG Fc Glycans in Inflammation

Antibody-mediated inflammatory responses are central in protection against infectious diseases and malignancies. While inflammatory effector functions can protect against disease, dysregulation of the response can result in autoimmunity or other pathologic inflammation. Balanced signaling through Type I and Type II FcγRs is required for moderation of inflammatory responses. This balance is achieved, in part, through regulated sialylation of Fc glycans, which is the determinant of binding to Type II FcγRs; it is based on the ability to interact with sialylated immune complexes that Type I and Type II FcγRs are distinguished. Fc sialylation has the effect of reducing binding to Type I FcγRs while enabling engagement of Type II FcγRs.

Increased Type II FcγR signaling due to the presence of sialylated Fc glycans can trigger potent anti-inflammatory activity. A classic example of this is observed with administration of high dose intravenous immunoglobulin (IVIg) during acute inflammatory diseases such as immune thrombocytopenia, Kawasaki disease, chronic inflammatory demyelinating polyneuropathy and Guillain-Barre syndrome. IVIg is pooled IgG from thousands of donors and its anti-inflammatory activity is mediated by the minor subset of IgGs within the pool that contain sialylated Fcs (Imbach et al. 1981; Debre et al. 1993; Kaneko et al. 2006). Anti-inflammatory activity can be increased by enhancing the abundance of sialylated Fcs within the IgG pool (Washburn et al. 2015). Sialylated Fcs in IVIg signal through the Type II FcγR DC-SIGN on regulatory macrophages leading to production of interleukin 33 (IL-33). IL-33, in turn, triggers release of IL-4 by basophils, resulting in increased FcγRIIb expression on effector myeloid cells, including monocytes and macrophages at sites of inflammation (Anthony et al. 2011; Schwab et al. 2012; Schwab et al. 2014). A recent study of in vivo sialylation by recombinantly produced glycosyltransferases found that increasing sialylation of endogenous IgG could treat autoimmune sequelae in a similar pathway that required DC-SIGN and FcγRIIb (Pagan et al. 2017). Regulated expression of FcγRIIb constitutes a powerful mechanism for controlling inflammation, with increased FcγRIIb expression elevating the threshold of cellular activation and effectively reducing the inflammatory response by these cells (Santiago-Raber et al. 2009; Dhodapkar et al. 2007; Kaneko et al. 2006; Boruchov et al. 2005; Lehmann et al. 2012). In addition to the DC-SIGN/FcγRIIb pathway, IL-33 release induced by administration of sialylated Fcs can trigger a potent regulatory T cell response that is sufficient to control T cell mediated inflammation in the experimental autoimmune encephalomyelitis model (Fiebiger et al. 2015). Fc glycan sialylation is thus a central regulator of inflammation. Interestingly, differences in baseline Fc sialylation among people can exceed 20% in health, a magnitude well within the range that is associated with changes in Type II FcγR-mediated processes and inflammatory activity (Wang et al. 2015; Pfeifle et al. 2016; Maamary et al. 2017; Fokkink et al. 2014). This implicates Fc sialylation as a driver of diversity in inflammatory thresholds among people.

Another mechanism by which IgG Fc glycoforms act in homeostatic regulation of inflammation involves the Type I FcγR, FcγRIIIa. This activating receptor is expressed on NK cells and subsets of monocytes and macrophages where it mediates activities including cell cytotoxicity, effector cell activation, inflammatory cytokine production and is a minor mediator of phagocytosis (relative to FcγRIIa) (Rafiq et al. 2013; Shalova et al. 2012; Yeap et al. 2016). Dysregulated FcγRIIIa activity is associated with pathologic sequelae such as alloantibody mediated diseases in neonates (Kapur et al. 2014; Sonneveld et al. 2016; Wuhrer et al. 2009) and progression to severe disease and autoimmune pathology during dengue infection. A critical mechanism for controlling signaling through FcγRIIIa in vivo is through regulation of Fc glycan fucosylation. Specifically, IgG1 Fc glycans lacking a core fucose residue (afucosylated Fc glycans) have higher affinity for FcγRIIIa (and FcγRIIIb) due to an unusual, stabilizing sugar–sugar interaction (Ferrara et al. 2011). While afucosylation impacts the affinity of both FcγRIIIa and FcγRIIIb, FcγRIIIb is expressed solely on neutrophils and lacks signaling capacity; thus, the major role of fucosylation on antibody activity is through modulation of FcγRIIIa binding. Afucosylated IgG1 antibodies have approximately 5-fold or 2-fold enhanced affinity for the low (F158) and high (V158) isoforms of FcγRIIIa, respectively.

The role of afucosylated Fc glycoforms in modulating inflammatory responses is well demonstrated in dengue infections, where antibodies play a direct role in mediating the severe forms of disease, dengue hemorrhagic fever and dengue shock syndrome. While anti-dengue antibodies can protect, they can also trigger progression to these severe disease states that cause a majority of dengue-associated deaths. Disease progression is largely mediated by virus particles that are bound by IgGs that don't neutralize the virus. Instead, the virus immune complexes increase virus infection and modulate cytokine production in FcγR-bearing cells (Halstead 2009). Risk for severe dengue is nearly doubled in individuals who produce high levels ($\geq 10\%$) of afucosylated Fc glycans, implicating FcγRIIIa in the pathogenesis of severe dengue (Wang et al. 2017). In healthy adults, afucosylated of IgG1 Fc glycans are nearly always found at levels <10% of all glycoforms but can reach >20% in some individuals. During actue dengue infections, afucosylation of IgG1 is elevated and can approach 30% in some individuals with severe disease (Wang et al. 2017).

One mechanism by which afucosylated IgGs impact dengue disease is through the activity of antibodies that cross-react between the dengue non-structural protein 1 (NS1) and a platelet antigen (Wan et al. 2016). Highly afucosylated anti-NS1 IgGs can mediate platelet loss in vivo, a defining feature of severe dengue disease. Aside from mediating platelet loss, increased afucosylated anti-dengue IgGs during acute infection correlate with increases in hematocrit, the hallmark of plasma leak which defines severe dengue (Wang et al. 2017). This association suggests an additional role for afucosylated Fc glycoforms and FcγRIIIa in severe dengue through an inflammatory cascade that results in vascular permeability. The role of afucosylated IgGs in dengue infection is a clear example of how the basal Fc glycoform repertoire can drive heterogeneity in human disease susceptibilities and outcomes.

4 IgG Fc Glycans and Adaptive Immunity

Immune complex interactions with FcγRs mediate several cellular processes involved in the maturation of high affinity antibody responses. These include: efficient transport of antigen to the germinal center, processing and presentation of antigens to T cells, and selection of B cells based on affinity of the B cell receptor (Wang et al. 2015; Regnault et al. 1999; Getahun et al. 2004; de Jong et al. 2006; Ding et al. 2016; Hjelm et al. 2008). The role of sialylated Fc glycans within immune complexes in B cell selection was recently discovered and involves a mechanism whereby Type I and Type II FcγRs act in cis to promote selection of B cells with high affinity B cell receptors (BCRs) (Wang et al. 2015; Maamary et al. 2017).

The mechanism by which sialylated Fc glycans impact B cell selection relies on the activity of FcγRIIb in regulating thresholds for B cell activation. Expression of activating Type I FcγRs is nearly always coupled to expression of the inhibitory Type I FcγRIIb; this combined expression ensures balanced signaling and is required by most leukocyte types for specificity of cellular maturation and effector activities (Boruchov et al. 2005; Clynes et al. 1999; Dhodapkar et al. 2005; McGaha et al. 2005). B cells represent an important exception to this rule as they express FcγRIIb throughout development, without co-expression of activating FcγRs. FcγRIIb on B cells acts to moderate the cell-activating signals that are triggered by antigen binding to the B cell receptor (BCR). Thus, a key variable in regulation of B cell activation is the expression level of FcγRIIb, which changes with development of B cells, but is also inducible. In the absence of inhibitory FcγRIIb or with low-level expression or signaling, B cells lack appropriate activation thresholds and produce higher titer, low avidity IgGs. The activation thresholds defined through FcγRIIb signaling are in fact required for maintenance of immune tolerance, with autoantibody production observed in FcγRIIb$^{-/-}$ mice and low levels of B cell FcγRIIb found in patients with autoantibody mediated diseases (McGaha et al. 2005; Fukuyama et al. 2005; Kono et al. 2005; Li et al. 2014; Su et al. 2004; Tackenberg et al. 2009; Mackay et al. 2006; Baerenwaldt et al. 2011). FcγRIIb signaling alone on B cells, as can occur in the presence of immune complexes formed from antigens that are not reactive with the BCR, induces pro-apoptotic signals. This pro-apoptotic signaling is attenuated by BCR engagement, ensuring preservation of cells that can respond to relevant antigens (Ono et al. 1997; Pearse et al. 1999).

As FcγRIIb is a critical determinant of B cell selection, regulation of its expression over time is essential. Temporal association of B cell FcγRIIb expression with the presence of antigen is achieved, in part, by regulation of Fc sialylation on antigen-specific IgGs. This was discovered in studies that characterized a shift towards sialylated Fc glycan production on anti-hemagglutinin (HA) IgGs by day 7 post influenza virus vaccination (Selman et al. 2012a; Wang et al. 2015). To determine the role of sialylated immune complexes on maturation of the vaccine response, experiments were done which found that sialylated immune complexes could act through the Type II FcγR, CD23, to induce increased expression of FcγRIIb on B cells. Elevated FcγRIIb, in turn, increases the threshold for activation of B cells that occurs with BCR signaling, resulting in selection of higher affinity, antigen-specific B cells. This mechanism can be recapitulated experimentally by administration of sialylated immune complexes to mice, leading to increased FcγRIIb on germinal center B cells and production of higher affinity antibodies in a CD23-dependent manner (Wang et al. 2015; Maamary et al. 2017). How other modulations in Fc glycoforms that occur following vaccination impact maturation of the vaccine response has yet to be discovered.

5 Heterogeneity and Regulation of Fc Glycoforms

While the regulators of Fc glycan modifications are not well understood, it is clear that multiple mechanisms impact the Fc glycoform repertoire in humans. One type of regulation is apparent at the level of antigen specificity. An example of this is observed in the antibody response against the influenza HA, in which anti-HA globular head IgGs are significantly more sialylated and fucosylated than stalk-reactive IgGs (Wang et al. 2015). Significant differences in IgG1 Fc sialylation are also observed between IgGs that react with H1 or H3 subtype HA glycoproteins (Wang, unpublished observation). Total IgG Fc glycans (all subclasses) also vary with Fab specificity when comparing IgGs reactive with different HIV proteins in infected individuals (Mahan et al. 2016). Other examples of correlations between Fc glycosylation and Fab specificity have been found in autoimmune diseases such as granulomatosis with polyangiitis (GPA) and rheumatoid arthritis (RA). These diseases are marked by the presence of autoantibodies such as anti—PR3 and anti-ACPA, found in GPA and RA respectively. Anti-PR3 and anti-ACPA can have reduced Fc sialylation over total IgG and may contribute to disease pathogenesis during disease flares through increased Type I FcγR-mediated cellular activation (Wuhrer et al. 2015; Kaneko et al. 2006; Scherer et al. 2010).

Distinctions in Fc glycosylation that are linked to Fab specificity are likely, in part, a consequence of selective glycosylation by different IgG-producing B cell subsets. This is supported by the finding that plasmablasts and memory B cells produce distinct amounts of ST6GAL1 and FUT8, the glycosyltransferases responsible for Fc sialylation and fucosylation, respectively (Wang et al. 2015). Expansion of plasmablasts, which express higher levels of ST6GAL1 and FUT8 in the days following vaccination, is mirrored by production of highly sialylated, fucosylated anti-HA IgGs. In contrast, anti-stalk IgGs, which are likely to be derived from the memory B cell pool, are modified by lower levels of Fc sialylation and fucosylation (Wang et al. 2015).

A second level of Fc glycan regulation occurs with the IgG subclass. Fc glycoforms are distinct depending on the IgG subclass with IgG1 trending toward lower sialylation and fucosylation than other subclasses (Wuhrer et al. 2015; Wang, unpublished observation). The activity of various Fc glycoforms on IgG2, IgG3 and IgG4 subclasses is not yet known however, so how this differential glycosylation contributes to immune homeostasis remains to be discovered.

In addition to differences in Fc glycosylation that occur with Fab specificity or IgG subclass, Fc glycan repertoires vary with the physiologic compartment from which the IgG was isolated. For example, IgGs from the cerebrospinal fluid of patients with multiple sclerosis have reduced sialylation compared with matched donor serum IgGs (Wuhrer et al. 2015). Another study found that Fc galactosylation, the precursor to sialylation, is reduced on synovial fluid IgGs relative to serum IgGs in RA patients (Scherer et al. 2010). The basis of differences in Fc glycosylation associated with physiologic compartments is not known but may involve production by distinct B cell subsets or variation in the availability of saccharide precursors.

While Fc glycan modifications are generally believed to occur within B cells, a topic of some debate is whether any sialylation of Fc glycans occurs extracellularly, in the absence of exogenously administered glycosyltrasferases (Jones et al. 2012, 2016). In favor of sialylation within B cells, human B cell ST6GAL1 and the abundance of sialylation on secreted IgGs can be modulated by cytokines present in cell culture (Selman et al. 2012a; Wang et al. 2011) or increased in vivo by estrogen treatment in postmenopausal patients with rheumatoid arthritis (Engdahl et al. 2018). In addition, human B cell ST6GAL1 expression correlates with Fc sialylation after vaccination (Wang et al. 2015). Another recent study showed that ST6Gal1 is regulated by IL-23 in antibody producing cells (APCs). This regulation was a consequence of IL-23 acting on TH17 cells which suppressed ST6Gal1 expression in an IL-21 and IL-22-dependent pathway (Pfeifle et al. 2016). Overall, data supporting an extracellular mechanism in humans have not yet been described but several factors implicate a dominant B cell intrinsic pathway.

Finally, an important variable among studies of Fc glycosylation in humans relates to the methods used for glycan measurement. In order to interpret data for sound hypothesis generation, the analysis should reflect the Fc domain repertoire that would be present in relevant immune complexes. This requires that the analysis be (1) antigen specific, (2) IgG subclass specific and (3) Fc domain specific. Antigen specific analysis is important because of the segregation of glycans by Fab specificity. Similarly, subclass specific analysis is critical because Fc glycoforms vary by subclass and because the activity of different glycoforms on IgG2, IgG3 and IgG4 antibodies is unknown, as discussed above. Thus, at this time, only data on IgG1 Fc glycosylation is truly interpretable for hypothesis generation. Importantly, bulk IgG glycan analysis cannot be used for hypothesis generation because of the lack of antigen and subclass specificity but also because approximately 20% of IgGs are glycosylated within their Fab domains and those glycoforms are entirely distinct in repertoire from those that modify the Fc (Mimura et al. 2007). Therefore, a detailed study of the methods used for glycan analysis is required of readers who wish to interpret published studies on IgG glycosylation.

6   Concluding Remarks

IgG Fc glycan modifications are a key regulator of antibody activity in vivo. While Fc sialylation has an active role in anti-inflammatory signaling and in maturation of adaptive immune responses, fucosylation of the Fc is regulated to drive appropriate pro-inflammatory effector cell functions. A critical question for future studies to address is how the human Fc glycoform repertoire is regulated. Understanding this will be necessary to shift endogenous Fc glycosylation for therapeutic benefit, which could potentially be done to treat diseases responsive to IVIg therapy, to enhance the activity of anti-tumor antibodies, to prevent autoantibody-mediated tissue disease, to enhance the quality of antibodies generated during vaccination or to reduce the mortality associated with dengue virus infections. The ability to direct shifts in the Fc domain repertoire, in both IgG subclass distribution and Fc glycosylation, is an exciting prospect for treating and preventing human diseases through tuning of the interaction between antibodies and their receptors.

Acknowledgements Support was received from Stanford University, the Chan Zuckerberg Biohub and the Searle Scholars Program. Research reported in this publication was supported in part by the Bill & Melinda Gates Foundation (OPP1188461) and the National Institutes of Health (1R01AI139119-01A1, 5K22AI12347802, 5U19AI111825-05, UL1TR001866).

References

Anthony RM et al (2011) Intravenous gammaglobulin suppresses inflammation through a novel T (H)2 pathway. Nature 475(7354):110–113

Baerenwaldt A et al (2011) Fcγ receptor IIB (FcγRIIB) maintains humoral tolerance in the human immune system in vivo. Proc Natl Acad Sci U S A 108(46):18772–18777

Barb AW, Brady EK, Prestegard JH (2009) Branch-specific sialylation of IgG-Fc glycans by ST6Gal-I. Biochemistry 48(41):9705–9707

Boruchov AM et al (2005) Activating and inhibitory IgG Fc receptors on human DCs mediate opposing functions. J Clin Invest 115(10):2914–2923

Clynes R et al (1999) Modulation of immune complex-induced inflammation in vivo by the coordinate expression of activation and inhibitory Fc receptors. J Exp Med 189(1):179–185

de Jong JM et al (2006) Dendritic cells, but not macrophages or B cells, activate major histocompatibility complex class II-restricted CD4$^+$ T cells upon immune-complex uptake in vivo. Immunology 119(4):499–506

Debre M et al (1993) Infusion of Fcγ fragments for treatment of children with acute immune thrombocytopenic purpura. Lancet 342(8877):945–949

Dhodapkar KM et al (2005) Selective blockade of inhibitory Fcγ receptor enables human dendritic cell maturation with IL-12p70 production and immunity to antibody-coated tumor cells. Proc Natl Acad Sci U S A 102(8):2910–2915

Dhodapkar KM et al (2007) Selective blockade of the inhibitory Fcγ receptor (FcγRIIB) in human dendritic cells and monocytes induces a type I interferon response program. J Exp Med 204 (6):1359–1369

Ding Z et al (2016) IgE-mediated enhancement of CD4(+) T cell responses requires antigen presentation by CD8α(-) conventional dendritic cells. Sci Rep 6:28290

Endy TP et al (2004) Relationship of preexisting dengue virus (DV) neutralizing antibody levels to viremia and severity of disease in a prospective cohort study of DV infection in Thailand. J Infect Dis 189(6):990–1000

Engdahl C et al (2018) Estrogen induces St6gal1 expression and increases IgG sialylation in mice and patients with rheumatoid arthritis: a potential explanation for the increased risk of rheumatoid arthritis in postmenopausal women. Arthritis Res Ther 20(1):84

Ferrara C et al (2006) Modulation of therapeutic antibody effector functions by glycosylation engineering: influence of Golgi enzyme localization domain and co-expression of heterologous β1, 4-N-acetylglucosaminyltransferase III and Golgi α-mannosidase II. Biotechnol Bioeng 93 (5):851–861

Ferrara C et al (2011) Unique carbohydrate–carbohydrate interactions are required for high affinity binding between FcγRIII and antibodies lacking core fucose. Proc Natl Acad Sci U S A 108 (31):12669–12674

Fiebiger BM et al (2015) Protection in antibody- and T cell-mediated autoimmune diseases by antiinflammatory IgG Fcs requires type II FcRs. Proc Natl Acad Sci U S A 112(18):E2385–E2394

Flynn GC et al (2010) Naturally occurring glycan forms of human immunoglobulins G1 and G2. Mol Immunol 47(11–12):2074–2082

Fokkink WJ et al (2014) IgG Fc N-glycosylation in Guillain-Barre syndrome treated with immunoglobulins. J Proteome Res 13(3):1722–1730

Fukuyama H, Nimmerjahn F, Ravetch JV (2005) The inhibitory Fcγ receptor modulates autoimmunity by limiting the accumulation of immunoglobulin G+ anti-DNA plasma cells. Nat Immunol 6(1):99–106

Getahun A et al (2004) IgG2a-mediated enhancement of antibody and T cell responses and its relation to inhibitory and activating Fcγ receptors. J Immunol 172(9):5269–5276

Halstead SB (2009) Antibodies determine virulence in dengue. Ann N Y Acad Sci 1171(Suppl 1): E48–E56

Hjelm F, Karlsson MC, Heyman B (2008) A novel B cell-mediated transport of IgE-immune complexes to the follicle of the spleen. J Immunol 180(10):6604–6610

Hodoniczky J, Zheng YZ, James DC (2005) Control of recombinant monoclonal antibody effector functions by Fc N-glycan remodeling in vitro. Biotechnol Prog 21(6):1644–1652

Imbach P et al (1981) High-dose intravenous gammaglobulin for idiopathic thrombocytopenic purpura in childhood. Lancet 1(8232):1228–1231

Jones MB et al (2012) Anti-inflammatory IgG production requires functional P1 promoter in β-galactoside α2,6-sialyltransferase 1 (ST6Gal-1) gene. J Biol Chem 287(19):15365–15370

Jones MB et al (2016) B-cell-independent sialylation of IgG. Proc Natl Acad Sci U S A 113 (26):7207–7212

Kaneko Y, Nimmerjahn F, Ravetch JV (2006a) Anti-inflammatory activity of immunoglobulin G resulting from Fc sialylation. Science 313(5787):670–673

Kaneko Y et al (2006b) Pathology and protection in nephrotoxic nephritis is determined by selective engagement of specific Fc receptors. J Exp Med 203(3):789–797

Kao D et al (2015) A monosaccharide residue is sufficient to maintain mouse and human IgG subclass activity and directs IgG effector functions to cellular Fc receptors. Cell Rep 13 (11):2376–2385

Kapur R et al (2014) A prominent lack of IgG1-Fc fucosylation of platelet alloantibodies in pregnancy. Blood 123(4):471–480

Kono H et al (2005) FcγRIIB Ile232Thr transmembrane polymorphism associated with human systemic lupus erythematosus decreases affinity to lipid rafts and attenuates inhibitory effects on B cell receptor signaling. Hum Mol Genet 14(19):2881–2892

Lehmann B et al (2012) FcγRIIB: a modulator of cell activation and humoral tolerance. Expert Rev Clin Immunol 8(3):243–254

Li F, Smith P, Ravetch JV (2014) Inhibitory Fcγ receptor is required for the maintenance of tolerance through distinct mechanisms. J Immunol 192(7):3021–3028

Lux A et al (2013) Impact of immune complex size and glycosylation on IgG binding to human FcγRs. J Immunol 190(8):4315–4323

Maamary J et al (2017) Increasing the breadth and potency of response to the seasonal influenza virus vaccine by immune complex immunization. Proc Natl Acad Sci U S A

Mackay M et al (2006) Selective dysregulation of the FcγIIB receptor on memory B cells in SLE. J Exp Med 203(9):2157–2164

Mahan AE et al (2015) A method for high-throughput, sensitive analysis of IgG Fc and Fab glycosylation by capillary electrophoresis. J Immunol Methods 417:34–44

Mahan AE et al (2016) Antigen-specific antibody glycosylation is regulated via vaccination. PLoS Pathog 12(3):e1005456

McGaha TL, Sorrentino B, Ravetch JV (2005) Restoration of tolerance in lupus by targeted inhibitory receptor expression. Science 307(5709):590–593

Mimura Y et al (2007) Contrasting glycosylation profiles between Fab and Fc of a human IgG protein studied by electrospray ionization mass spectrometry. J Immunol Methods 326(1–2):116–126

Ono M et al (1997) Deletion of SHIP or SHP-1 reveals two distinct pathways for inhibitory signaling. Cell 90(2):293–301

Pagan JD, Kitaoka M, Anthony RM (2017) Engineered sialylation of pathogenic antibodies in vivo attenuates autoimmune disease. Cell

Pearse RN et al (1999) SHIP recruitment attenuates FcγRIIB-induced B cell apoptosis. Immunity 10(6):753–760

Pfeifle R et al (2016) Regulation of autoantibody activity by the IL-23-TH17 axis determines the onset of autoimmune disease. Nat Immunol

Rafiq S et al (2013) Comparative assessment of clinically utilized CD20-directed antibodies in chronic lymphocytic leukemia cells reveals divergent NK cell, monocyte, and macrophage properties. J Immunol 190(6):2702–2711

Regnault A et al (1999) Fcgamma receptor-mediated induction of dendritic cell maturation and major histocompatibility complex class I-restricted antigen presentation after immune complex internalization. J Exp Med 189(2):371–380

Santiago-Raber ML et al (2009) Fcγ receptor-dependent expansion of a hyperactive monocyte subset in lupus-prone mice. Arthritis Rheum 60(8):2408–2417

Scherer HU et al (2010) Glycan profiling of anti-citrullinated protein antibodies isolated from human serum and synovial fluid. Arthritis Rheum 62(6):1620–1629

Schwab I et al (2012) IVIg-mediated amelioration of ITP in mice is dependent on sialic acid and SIGNR1. Eur J Immunol 42(4):826–830

Schwab I et al (2014) Broad requirement for terminal sialic acid residues and FcγRIIB for the preventive and therapeutic activity of intravenous immunoglobulins in vivo. Eur J Immunol 44(5):1444–1453

Selman MH et al (2012a) Changes in antigen-specific IgG1 Fc N-glycosylation upon influenza and tetanus vaccination. Mol Cell Proteomics 11(4):M111 014563

Selman MH et al (2012b) Fc specific IgG glycosylation profiling by robust nano-reverse phase HPLC-MS using a sheath-flow ESI sprayer interface. J Proteomics 75(4):1318–1329

Shalova IN et al (2012) CD16 regulates TRIF-dependent TLR4 response in human monocytes and their subsets. J Immunol 188(8):3584–3593

Shinkawa T et al (2003) The absence of fucose but not the presence of galactose or bisecting N-acetylglucosamine of human IgG1 complex-type oligosaccharides shows the critical role of enhancing antibody-dependent cellular cytotoxicity. J Biol Chem 278(5):3466–3473

Sonneveld ME et al (2016) Glycosylation pattern of anti-platelet IgG is stable during pregnancy and predicts clinical outcome in alloimmune thrombocytopenia. Br J Haematol 174(2):310–320

Su K et al (2004) A promoter haplotype of the immunoreceptor tyrosine-based inhibitory motif-bearing FcγRIIb alters receptor expression and associates with autoimmunity. I. Regulatory FCGR2B polymorphisms and their association with systemic lupus erythematosus. J Immunol 172(11):7186–7191

Tackenberg B et al (2009) Impaired inhibitory Fcγ receptor IIB expression on B cells in chronic inflammatory demyelinating polyneuropathy. Proc Natl Acad Sci U S A 106(12):4788–4792

Wan SW et al (2016) Anti-dengue virus nonstructural protein 1 antibodies contribute to platelet phagocytosis by macrophages. Thromb Haemost 115(3):646–656

Wang J et al (2011) Fc-glycosylation of IgG1 is modulated by B-cell stimuli. Mol Cell Proteomics 10(5):M110 004655

Wang TT et al (2015) Anti-HA glycoforms drive B cell affinity selection and determine influenza vaccine efficacy. Cell 162(1):160–169

Wang TT et al (2017) IgG antibodies to dengue enhanced for FcγRIIIA binding determine disease severity. Science 355(6323):395–398

Washburn N et al (2015) Controlled tetra-Fc sialylation of IVIg results in a drug candidate with consistent enhanced anti-inflammatory activity. Proc Natl Acad Sci U S A

Wuhrer M et al (2009) Regulated glycosylation patterns of IgG during alloimmune responses against human platelet antigens. J Proteome Res 8(2):450–456

Wuhrer M et al (2015a) Skewed Fc glycosylation profiles of anti-proteinase 3 immunoglobulin G1 autoantibodies from granulomatosis with polyangiitis patients show low levels of bisection, galactosylation, and sialylation. J Proteome Res 14(4):1657–1665

Wuhrer M et al (2015b) Pro-inflammatory pattern of IgG1 Fc glycosylation in multiple sclerosis cerebrospinal fluid. J Neuroinflammation 12:235

Yeap WH et al (2016) CD16 is indispensable for antibody-dependent cellular cytotoxicity by human monocytes. Sci Rep 6:34310

IgE Glycosylation in Health and Disease

Kai-Ting Shade, Michelle E. Conroy and Robert M. Anthony

Contents

Abstract IgE are absolutely required for initiation of allergy reactions, which affect over 20% of the world's population. IgE are the least prevalent immunoglobulins in circulation with 12-h and 2-day half-lives in mouse and human serum, respectively, but an extended tissue half-life of 3-weeks bound to the surface of mast cells by the high affinity IgE receptor, FcεRI (Gould and Sutton 2008). Although the importance of glycosylation to IgG biology is well established, less is known regarding the contribution of IgE glycosylation to allergic inflammation. IgE has seven and nine N-linked glycosylation sites distributed across human and murine constant chains, respectively. Here we discuss studies that have analyzed IgE glycosylation and its function, and how IgE glycosylation contributions to health and disease.

1   IgE Biology in Health and Disease

IgE antibody induced inflammation is nearly synonymous with allergic disease, which affects one in five individuals worldwide. IgE are central to the mechanisms of immediate type hypersensitivity reactions. These antibodies are also somewhat enigmatic given that a comprehensive understanding of IgE biology has yet to be

K.-T. Shade · M. E. Conroy · R. M. Anthony (✉)
Massachusetts General Hospital, Center for Immunology and Inflammatory Diseases,
Harvard Medical School, 149 13th Street, Room 8.321, Boston, MA 02129, USA
e-mail: Robert.Anthony@mgh.harvard.edu

Current Topics in Microbiology and Immunology (2019) 423: 77–94
https://doi.org/10.1007/82_2019_151
© Springer Nature Switzerland AG 2019
Published online: 01 March 2019

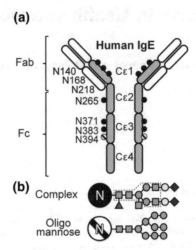

Fig. 1 Human IgE and its glycans. a Schematics of IgE structure and glycosylation. Predicted N-glycosylation sites in each constant domain (Cε) are represented by closed and open circles for complex and oligomannose glycans, respectively. **b** Complex glycans are composed of fucose (red), GlcNAc (blue), mannose (green), galactose (yellow circles), and sialic acid (pink). Core complex structure is shown in dotted box. Oligomannose glycans are composed of GlcNAc and between 5 and 9 mannoses

established. IgE antibodies are the subclass found least in the serum compared to IgM, IgG and IgA, with a concentration of 50–100 ng/ml, markedly lower than IgG (5–10 mg/ml). Compared to its long tissue half life of weeks, IgE serum half life is only 2–3 days (Vieira and Rajewsky 1988). Structurally, it differs from IgG in that it contains four domains in the constant region (Cε1-4, Fig. 1a) compared to three in IgG (Gould et al. 2003). In the constant domains, receptor binding occurs, yielding IgE effector functions. The IgE receptor, FcεRI, has strikingly high affinity for the antibody, $\sim 10^{11} \text{ M}^{-1}$, and is the source of the long tissue phase of IgE (Chang 2000). FcεRI coats the surface of cells including mast cells, basophils, as well as dendritic cells, Langerhans cells and eosinophils in humans. Notably, there are structural variations in FcεRI present in these cell types which result in differential effects upon binding. Mast cells and basophils express FcεRI as a tetramer, $\alpha\beta\gamma_2$, with the α unit responsible for IgE binding at the Cε3 domain. The β chain of the receptor is mainly responsible for signal amplification and is notably absent in the trimeric form of FcεRI, $\alpha\gamma_2$ present on dendritic cells, Langerhan cells, and eosniphils. The γ subunit is critical as it is the main structure responsible for orchestrating intra-cellular signaling pathways (Kraft and Kinet 2007). Allergen binding to IgE and subsequent cross linking of FcεRI receptors activates ITAMs and subsequent downstream signaling. Specifically, FcεRI is responsible for the canonical symptoms of immediate type hypersensitivity reactions detailed below.

There is a second IgE receptor, known as both CD23 and FcεRII. This is often referred to as the "low affinity" receptor given that the affinity coefficient, 10^6–10^7 M^{-1}, is dwarfed by that of FcεRI. This immunoglobulin receptor has a trimeric C-type lectin like globular domains extracellularly, one transmembrane domain and a short cytoplasmic domain. Interestingly, CD23 can be either membrane bound or soluble forms. CD23 is expressed across a variety of cells including T and B lymphocytes, follicular dendritic cells, and epithelial cells (Armitage et al. 1989; Rieber 1993; Yu et al. 2003). Upon activation, membrane bound CD23 causes suppression of IgE production by B cells. Secreted CD23 can exist in monomeric or trimeric structures and can either down or up-regulate IgE synthesis, depending of its oligomerization (McCloskey et al. 2007). Taken together, CD23 is a potent factor in maintaining IgE homeostasis. Additional cells including antigen-presenting and gut epithelial cells utilize CD23 for transcytosis cross epithelial barriers and subsequent allergen presentation to the immune system (Palaniyandi et al. 2011).

As mentioned above, IgE antibodies are present in very low levels in the serum, particularly compared to other immunoglobulin subclasses. This suggests that control of IgE production is very tightly regulated. After initial and successful VDJ recombination yields a functional B cell receptor, production of eventually IgE occurs as a result of IgM+ and IgD+ B cell activation. Tissue Th2 cells as well as Tfh and Th2-like cells in lymphoid organs have been identified as possible sources of cytokines to promote B cell preferential class switch to IgE (Reinhardt et al. 2009). Class switch recombination (CSR) to IgE is triggered upon ligation of CD40, activation of certain toll like receptors and BAFF in the context of IL-4 exposure (Geha et al. 2003). Transcription promoters lie just upstream of DNA switch (S) regions and are responsible for "selection" of particular S recombinations and resultant specific antibody subclass production. In the case of IgE, ligation of the IL-4 receptor triggers STAT6 activation which is phosphorylated and translocates to the nucleus, binding the IgE promoter (Hebenstreit et al. 2006). For counter-regulation, Bcl-6 can bind sites in the IgE promoter which overlap with STAT6 binding loci, leading to inhibition of IgE class switch (Harris 1999). Notably, class switch to IgE can occur in two possible ways- direct switch from IgM to IgE or IgM to IgG and finally IgE. In B cells stimulated by IL4 and LPS, IgG1 was produced initially and IgE several hours later (Mandler 1993). Wesemann et al. then showed similar sequential production in the context of IL4 and anti-CD40 stimulation (Wesemann et al. 2011). Preferential class switch between IgG and IgE is determined by various factors. Intriguingly, the IgG1 switch region contains the most target sequences for AID, the enzyme responsible for class switching, and IgE the fewest. The IgG1 switch region may also block accessibility to the IgE S region (Misaghi et al. 2013) and accessibility to the IgE S region also seems to occur with a delayed rate (Wesemann et al. 2012). Taken together, control of class switching to IgE is an important means through which the antibody level can be tightly controlled. In addition, and critically, sequential class switch to IgE results in high-affinity antibody, perhaps owing to the longer timeline and persistent exposure to AID, also responsible for affinity maturation. Direct class switch from IgM directly to IgE results in lower affinity antibodies (He et al. 2015). This has significant functional repercussions.

When considering where and when IgE class switch recombination, production and memory occur there are some puzzling curiosities. First and foremost, there seems to be an overall lack of IgE memory B cells found in immunologic tissues (Yang, Sullivan, and Allen 2012). Typically, in lymphoid germinal centers (GCs), B cell proliferation occurs with concurrent affinity maturation and positive selection via interactions with follicular dendritic cells and Tfh cells. Therefore, GC interactions are critical for the eventual development of memory B cells and plasma cells resulting in long lived antibody memory (Janeway et al. 2001). Murine studies demonstrated while IgE+ B cells were not found in spleen or lymph nodes, plasma cells represented the preponderance of IgE producing cells in these animals. These cells were noted to have undergone sequential switching, with an IgG intermediate, followed by rapid differentiation to IgE expressing plasma cells (Erazo et al. 2007). He et al. were able to show that GC IgE$^+$ cells do exist but that they expressed significantly lower expression of surface antibody, weak BCR signaling and did not populate GC light zone. This suggested that IgE$^+$ cells in germinal centers were dying prematurely in the maturation process (He et al. 2013). As noted previously, sequential class switching from IgG to IgE seems to provide the most significant source of high affinity antibody. Thus, IgG$^+$ B cells have been hypothesized as the source of IgE memory. B220$^+$ CD138$^-$IgG1$^+$ B cells have been identified as the cell population responsible for significant IgE memory production (He et al. 2013). Further, the same group identified a murine IgG1 memory B cell subset which was able to generate IgE$^+$ plasma cells and produce high affinity, functional antibody, able to trigger anaphylaxis in a murine model (He et al. 2017). Therefore, IgG$^+$ B cells serve as a main reservoir for IgE memory along with IgE$^+$ plasma cells. It is notable that direct class switch from IgM to IgE results in low affinity antibody production and short lived GC IgE$^+$ cells. Together, these cells and mechanisms are the source of both high and low affinity IgE antibodies and maintain the functional pool of IgE (He et al. 2015).

IgE antibodies have gained significant attention as the incidence of allergic diseases has increased substantially. The World Allergy Organization estimates that a staggering 30–40% of the world's population suffers from one or more allergic conditions (Pawankar et al. 2011). This contributes to substantial burden of illness and the economic implications are massive, thought to cost billions of dollars in medical visits and lost productivity (2010). Atopic diseases are considered to be one of the principle manifestations of IgE driven pathology. As discussed above, allergen specific IgE antibodies are bound to the surface of mast cells and basophils via Fc binding to the FcεRI receptor. Allergen cross linking of cell bound IgE results in cellular degranulation and canonical symptoms of allergic inflammation. Immediate release of mediators causes rapid onset of vascular dilation and permeability, bronchoconstriction, leukocyte extravasation and smooth muscle contraction. Cellular activation also results in synthetic processes which generate mediators of "late phase" reactions (Holgate 1982). These processes result in clinical symptoms including potentially fatal anaphylaxis. Allergen specific IgE can be utilized for diagnostics in allergy and is a target of therapies in asthma, environmental/food/venom allergies and atopic dermatitis.

Yet, significant IgE biology extends beyond allergic inflammation and atopic diseases. It has been implicated in protection against parasitic infection and venom exposures. Additionally, several non-allergic diseases also have IgE implicated in their pathogenesis. As previously described, IgE antibodies coat the surface of mast cells via the FcεRI receptor. Mast cells localize to vascularized tissues and are especially concentrated at mucosal and skin surfaces (Gurish and Austen 2012). In the context of parasitic infections, both parasite specific and non-specific IgE antibodies markedly increase (Anthony et al. 2007). There is speculation that these increased IgE levels may trigger mast cell activation at mucosal surfaces leading to various biologic functions which ultimately lead to worm expulsion. In general, specific mechanisms responsible for these actions are not well elucidated (Fitzsimmons et al. 2014). In fact, in mice infected with *Schistosoma mansoni*, significant manipulations of IgE levels did not specifically modulate host pathology from infection, though may have contributed to liver pathology (Jankovic 1997). The specific biologic relevance of IgE with regard to parasitic immunity remains to be deciphered.

As they are in parasitic diseases, mast cells are also felt to confer innate protection against toxic proteins such as those from insects and snakes. In murine models, venom proteins administered in vivo trigger mast cells to release pre-formed heparin that contribute to toxin neutralization (Mukai et al. 2016). Mast cell proteases have also been shown to directly reduce toxicity of venoms (Metz et al. 2006). Specific IgE antibodies against insect venoms are used as diagnostic tools to identify persons allergic to these proteins who may be at risk of anaphylaxis with subsequent exposures. It has therefore been presumed that anti-venom IgE antibodies are pathogenic. However, with consideration of mast cell protective functions in the context of toxin exposures, several groups have questioned whether venom specific IgE may play a role in facilitating mast cell protective responses. Mice immunized with whole bee venom generated both IgG1 and IgE venom specific antibodies. Immunized mice were more resistant to subsequent exposure to lethal dosing of the same venom. IgE deficient and FcεRI$^{-/-}$ mice did not demonstrate this same resistance. Passive immunization with bee venom antibody containing serum also provided protection upon bee venom administration in IgE deficient mice (Marichal et al. 2013). In mice who were administered repeated immunization with phospholipase A2, known to be a potent allergenic component of honeybee venom, protection was established against subsequent lethal honeybee venom. This protection did not occur in mice who were B cell deficient or in those with dysfunctional FcεRI (Palm et al. 2013). Given that most humans with venom specific IgE have never had anaphylaxis in the context of exposure, Mukai et al. speculate that improved protection against venomous exposures may be an "ancient and fundamental" function of IgE and mast cells (Mukai et al. 2016).

IgE has largely been implicated in allergic diseases. However, their presence in diseases primarily involving immune system dysregulation have raised questions as to a more global immunologic role for IgE antibodies. As an example, decades ago, self-reactive IgE antibodies and IgE containing immune complexes were found in patients with systemic lupus erythematosus (SLE) (Miyawaki S 1973). It has been well established that self reactive immune complexes lead to production of type I interferons by plasmacytoid dendritic cells in SLE (Ronnblom 2001). Recently, Henault et al. demonstrated that the presence of DNA-IgE autoantibodies in human SLE caused self-DNA triggered TLR9 activation in plasmacytoid dendritic cells facilitated by the interaction of IgE/FcεRI. This lead to markedly increased production of IFN-α (Henault et al. 2016). They speculate that self dsDNA-IgE complexes may contribute to increased loss of tolerance and exacerbation of pathology as a result. In fact, higher levels of self-reactive dsDNA-IgE in the serum correlated with disease severity.

Immune deficiencies provide another clinical example in which IgE is elevated in the context of immune dysregulation. Hyper-IgE (HIES) or Job syndrome is a complex disease in which IgE levels can reach levels of more than 20,000 IU/L, orders of magnitude higher than normal (Sowerwine et al. 2012). The disease presents with a mysterious combination of symptoms including *Staph aureus* abscesses, eczematous rashes, recurrent sinopulmonary infections, chronic candida infections, eosinophilia, fungal infections, and EBV and VZV infections (Siegel et al. 2011). Notably, patients with HIES also present with osseous abnormalities including craniofacial dysmorphology, delayed tooth eruption and high arched palate (Nieminen et al. 2011). Malignancy affects significant numbers of these people as well, involving both blood and solid organs. These clinical manifestations are the result of STAT3 mutations on chromosome 17. This leads to abnormalities in the IL-6 pathway (Holland et al. 2007) and, significantly, marked inhibition of the Th17 immunologic response (Milner et al. 2008). The specific mechanisms responsible for the marked elevation in IgE levels is not fully known. Interestingly, Liu et al. recently showed that STAT3 deletion in keratinocytes of mice with eczema-like inflammation surprisingly lead to a marked elevation in IgE levels (Liu 2017). Cutaneous inflammation in this model was induced by *S. aureus*, which is also responsible for significant disease pathology in patients with HIES. Other immune deficiencies including DOCK8 deficiency, TYK2 deficiency, Omenn's syndrome, Wisoctt-Aldrich syndrome, DiGeorge syndrome, Netherton and IPEX syndromes have elevated IgE as a hallmark (Mogensen 2016). Once again, how IgE occurs in and affects these conditions is poorly understood and studies are ongoing to improve understanding.

2   IgE Structure

IgE and IgG are perhaps the most clinically relevant immunoglobulin classes. Further, there are a number of superficial similarities shared between these two molecules. Both are monomeric immunoglobulins comprised of two identical heavy chains and two identical light chains, and exert their canonical effector functions through interactions with Fc receptors expressed by innate cells. IgE heavy chains have four constant domains, and a single variable domain, and light chain has single constant and variable domains. Both IgE and IgG have been shown to adopt open and closed structures, that result in different Fc receptor binding profiles. While a single N-linked glycosylation site is present in all IgG, IgE is the most heavily glycosylated monomeric antibody.

Seven N-linked glycosylation sites are distributed across the constant domains of the human IgE heavy chains, while 9 sites are found on mouse IgE (Fig. 1a). One site, at asparagine (N) 394 on human IgE, is conserved across all mammalian IgE. The glycan that occupies the conserved site has an oligomannose structure (Fig. 1a, b). Indeed, this site is reported to be orthologous to the IgG glycosylation site (Wurzburg et al. 2000). Indeed, crystal structure of IgE and IgG Fcs feature a glycan, which is consist with glycans having a fixed position in the molecule. On human IgE, the remaining sites barring N383, which is unoccupied, contain mono- and di-sialylated complex biantennary glycans. Indeed, the published data on IgE from allergic patients is currently lacking, as analysis are restricted to IgE from serum of non-atopic (Plomp et al. 2013), hyperimmune (Arnold et al. 2004; Plomp et al. 2013), IgE myeloma (Plomp et al. 2013), and hyper IgE (Wu et al. 2016) patients, and recombinant sources (Shade et al. 2015). The IgE molecule adopts a bent horseshoe structure, where the Fab and Fc domains are folded towards each other. Further, the IgE Fab is rigid, unlike the flexible IgG hinge. It is thought the IgE molecule can rotate around it central axis reciprocally refolding. To date, no studies have detected the presence of O-linked glycosylation in IgE (Arnold et al. 2004; Plomp et al. 2013; Wu et al. 2016).

3 IgE N394 Glycosylation Site and Oligomannose Glycan

Important structural studies have revealed that IgE binds to FcεRI at the Cε3 domains and CD23 at both Cε3 and Cε4 domains of the Fc (Garman et al. 2000; Holdom et al. 2011). The interaction to each receptor is dependent on IgE conformation and is mutually exclusive, with FcεRI binding IgE in an open and CD23 in a closed conformation. The changes in conformation upon binding to one receptor disables binding to the other receptor. Over the past decade, strategies to alleviate IgE-mediated allergic diseases have generally been devised to prevent IgE-FcεRI interaction. This includes an anti-IgE therapeutic antibody Omalizumab that binds to an epitope overlapping FcεRI and directly prevents binding of serum free IgE to FcεRI. Another engineered protein inhibitor, designed ankyrin repeat protein (DARPin E2_79) also binds to the Cε3 and accelerates the dissociation of IgE from FcεRI on preformed complexes through an allosteric mechanism (Kim et al. 2012). Recently, a single-domain antibody derived from llama, sdab 026, have shown to inhibit IgE-FcεRI interaction by locking IgE in a closed conformation similar to CD23 binding and prevents the open conformation that allows the FcεRI interaction (Jabs et al. 2018).

Crystal structures of human IgE Fc also showed the glycans attached to N394 on the Cε3 domains occupy the cavity between two Fcs. This glycosylation site is evolutionary conserved across mammalian species and homologous to the key glycan attached on the IgG Fc (Jabs et al. 2018; Holdom et al. 2011; Wan et al. 2002; Garman et al. 2000; Sondermann et al. 2000). Previous studies have shown that IgG Fc glycans are critical for maintaining antibody structural conformation.

Removal of the Fc glycans results in a more closed conformation in the IgG Fcs and forfeits the functional conformation important for Fcγ receptor binding (Krapp et al. 2003; Feige et al. 2009). In comparison, conflicting studies between 1980 and early 2000 that used aglycosylated IgE produced from *Escherichia coli* or deglycosylated IgE or IgE Fc after enzymatic treatments make it hard to determine whether glycosylation modulates IgE functions.

The earliest studies using *E. coli*–derived recombinant IgE Fc or Cε3 domains revealed that aglycosylated IgE binds to FcεRI and can elicit IgE-mediated inflammation (Helm et al. 1998a, b; Henry et al. 2000). However, these proteins require additional manipulation including solubilization and refolding after recovery from bacterial insoluble inclusion bodies, which may compromise the native state of conformation. Later studies using enzymes to deglycosylate IgE Fc produced from mammalian cell lines or IgE derived from myeloma or serum showed incoherent results. While one study showed that deglycosylated IgE Fc retained binding to FcεRI with minimal difference in a radioligand competition binding assay (Basu et al. 1993), another showed a 4-fold lower binding affinity to FcεRI by SPR (Hunt et al. 2005). These results deviated from another study that showed significant impairment to FcεRI binding upon enzymatic deglycosylation (Bjorklund et al. 1999, 2000). On the other hand, all studies that genetically disrupted the N-linked glycosylation site N394 on IgE or IgE Fc by mutating asparagine-394 to glutamine (N394Q) or threonine (N394T), or alternatively disrupting the site by substituting the third amino acid in the Asn-X-Ser/Thr sequon theronine-396 to alanine (T396A), all abolished FcεRI binding and the subsequent IgE-mediated degranulation (Sayers et al. 1998; Shade et al. 2015; Jabs et al. 2018).

The functional significance of the glycan on IgE Fc was further exemplified by the in vivo work using mouse models (Shade et al. 2015) The equivalent of N394 is N384 in mouse. In mouse, genetic mutation (N384Q or T386A) or enzymatic digestion of IgE by PNG to remove all N-glycans lost the ability to bind FcεRI in vivo in ear mast cells and in vitro in ELISA or cell-based binding assays. As expected, IgE lacking N384 glycans were also unable to initiate immediate anaphylaxis in a passive cutaneous anaphylaxis mouse model. In a reciprocal experiment where all N-linked glycosylation sites were mutated except N384 (N384 only), this IgE was still able to elicit anaphylactic response similar to the WT, demonstrating that the glycan on the conserved site in IgE Fc is absolutely critical for IgE effector functions.

In contrast to the complex-type glycans on IgG Fc, all studies including crystal structure and glycopeptide mass spectrometry, uniformly identified the glycan attached to N394 is of oligomannose structures, with 2-9 mannose residues attached to two GlcNAc and $Man_5GlcNAc_2$ being the major form. IgE were sourced from monoclonal myeloma-derived, recombinant from different mammalian cell lines, serum of non-diseased donors, and serum of patients with hyperimmune conditions, IgE myeloma, atopic dermatitis or hyper IgE syndrome (Dorrington and Bennich 1978; Wan et al. 2002; Arnold et al. 2004; Holdom et al. 2011; Plomp et al. 2013; Shade et al. 2015; Wu et al. 2016). N-linked glycans of secreted mammalian proteins are typically processed to an intermediate oligomannose structure before further processed to hybrid and complex glycans in the lumen of the ER and the

Golgi. As mentioned, all other N-linked sites of IgE are composed of complex glycans. Thus, it is unique for glycans at N394 to retain the oligomannose structures from being converted to complex type. The mouse IgE homologue also harbors oligomannose glycans at the conserved site.

The functional significance of glycans at N394 and its exclusive composition of oligomannose structures provide a unique therapeutic opportunity to target this glycan. Unlike some of the other glycosidases that cleave all types of N-linked glycans, Endoglycosidase F1 selectively hydrolyses the oligomannose and hybrid structures and leaves complex structures unaffected. Mirroring genetically disruption of N394 glycosylation site on IgE, EndoF1-treated recombinant or native allergic human IgE lost its ability to bind FcεRI-expressed cells and elicit degranulation in mast cells. Mouse IgE digested with EndoF1 was also unable to initiate anaphylaxis in vivo (Shade et al. 2015). Being buried in the interstitial space between Fcs, the importance of N394 glycan is likely to maintain IgE protein structure as IgG glycans (Feige et al. 2009). Circular dichroism that measures the secondary structure of proteins revealed a shift in spectrum upon the loss of oligomannose glycans in IgE after EndoF1 treatment, reflecting changes in IgE three-dimensional conformation (Shade et al. 2015). This change likely explains the loss of functional protein folding necessary to bind FcεRI and initiate allergic inflammation.

In contrast to the requirement of IgE glycans in FcεRI interaction, deglycosylated myeloma IgE was reported to augment binding to CD23 on B cells (Vercelli et al. 1989). This finding reinforces the idea that IgE conformation decides the exclusive interaction with FcεRI or CD23. Perhaps the loss of glycans on IgE leads to a more closed conformation, thus promoting CD23 and preventing FcεRI binding.

4 Other N-Linked Glycosylation Sites on IgE

IgE is one of the most heavily glycosylated antibody class. Besides N394, IgE has six other glycosylation sites, of which five are known to have complex glycans attached (Fig. 1a, b). While oligomannose glycans are composed of only GlcNAc and mannose residues, complex glycans have additional sugars including fucose that attaches to the core structure and galactose or sialic acid to the terminal. To date, studies that described complex glycans on human recombinant, myeloma-derived or native IgE all revealed fucosylated sialylated structures to be the major complex glycoforms (Dorrington and Bennich 1978; Arnold et al. 2004; Plomp et al. 2013; Shade et al. 2015; Wu et al. 2016). Previous study has reported that deglycosylated IgE has a propensity to form aggregate (Basu et al. 1993). Thus, glycans on IgE probably contribute significantly to the water solubility of IgE and removal of these hydrophilic, acidic glycans may increase exposure of hydrophobic regions and results in aggregation. Various studies that mutated glycosylation sites with complex glycans attached in IgE Fc have thus far suggested a minimal role in IgE- FcεRI interaction. IgE/IgE Fc with single or double mutations at N265 and N374 sites was still able to bind FcεRI with the same affinity as the WT and initiate degranulation

(Nettleton and Kochan 1995; Young et al. 1995; Sayers et al. 1998; Shade et al. 2015). Interestingly, mutation of all N-linked sites in Cε1 domain of Fab portion showed a slight reduction in IgE-mediate degranulation (Shade et al. 2015), suggesting perhaps complex glycans in Cε1 modulates IgE interaction with the antigen.

Genetic disruption of the glycosylation site removes the entire glycan structure and disregards the roles that are dependent on the heterogeneity of the complex glycans. Studies of the complex glycans on IgG Fc demonstrated that these glycans are heterogeneous and can display more than 30 different glycoforms at a single site in healthy individuals (Kaneko et al. 2006; Wuhrer et al. 2007). These glycoforms reflect physiological processes and differ in diseases, serving as potential disease biomarkers. For example, changes in sialylation of IgG autoantibodies have been associated with clinical manifestation of the autoimmune and inflammatory diseases (Matsumoto et al. 2000; van de Geijn et al. 2009; Scherer et al. 2010; Ackerman et al. 2013a, b). Importantly, changes in glycoforms markedly modulate protein functions. When IgG is equipped with sialic acid, IgG shifts its receptor binding preferences and mediates anti-inflammatory activity (Kaneko et al. 2006; Anthony et al. 2008; Sondermann et al. 2013; Pincetic et al. 2014). Further, IgG that lack fucose has enhanced antibody-dependent cellular cytotoxicity as a result of increased affinity to FcγRIIIA by 50-fold (Shields et al. 2002; Ferrara et al. 2011).

In comparison to IgG, the role of complex glycans in IgE is not known. Studies of the ß-galactoside-binding lectins, galectins, have perhaps suggested the involvement of complex glycans in IgE-mediated functions. Galectin-3 has been shown to bind mouse IgE and activate IgE-sensitized rat basophilic leukemia cells (Frigeri et al. 1993; Liu et al. 1993; Zuberi et al. 1994). On the other hand, another galectin, galectin-9, has been shown to reduce mast cell degranulation and passive anaphylaxis by binding to IgE and inhibit its interaction with antigen (Niki et al. 2009). It is likely that these galectins bind to the complex glycans on the IgE to exert its regulatory roles. However, it is not clear how these two lectins work together in vivo, for example, whether they bind to the same glycans on IgE and their relevance in human physiology.

5 Conclusions and Future Perspectives

Despite its discovery over 50 years ago, much remains to be discovered relating to IgE. As mentioned above, it is not clear precisely what makes allergen-specific IgE pathogenic in some individuals, and inert in other. However, their role in diseases of intense public health interest mandate ongoing pursuit of a comprehensive rendering of their function and regulation. IgE is the most heavily glycosylated monomeric antibody, and the conserved glycan at N394 has an important role in conformational folding and binding to FcεRI. This work is in early stages and dedication to continued unraveling of the story is critical. However, even in these early stages of understanding, it is interesting to speculate as to how glycosylation could be a major factor in treatment of IgE-associated diseases in the future. As described previously, galectins may play a significant role in connecting IgE to its downstream effector functions. Recent studies have identified a role for Galectin-3 in the regulation of the IgE receptor, FcεRI. Utilizing RNAi screening experiments, one group recently demonstrated Gal-3 as a negative regulator of FcεRI triggered mast cell degranulation. Their data suggests Gal-3 may affect surface FcεRI internalization, receptor mobility, F-actin polymerization, and FcεRI ubiquination, all of which would profoundly impact mast cell signaling (Bambouskova et al. 2016). As altered variability in IgE glycosylation may impact galectin binding, it is certainly notable that activating or blocking interactions could yield substantial impact on the FcεRI and mast cell function. This would have marked impact on allergic inflammation. As a notable clinical correlate, Galectin-3 has been increasingly identified as a biomarker in various allergic diseases. A recent study identified Gal-3 as a marker increased in eosinophilic asthma but notably decreased in neutrophilic asthma (Gao et al. 2015). This finding was extended by Riccio et al. demonstrating Gal-3 as a predictive marker for positive response to anti-IgE treatment of asthma. Subjects positive for Gal-3 at baseline had more improvement in bronchial wall thickening, eosinophilic inflammation, and smooth muscle involvement (Riccio et al. 2017). Beyond asthma, a specific Gal-3 polymorphism has recently been identified as a significant genetic predictor of allergy to beta-lactam antibiotics (Cornejo-Garcia et al. 2016). These examples provide early clinical evidence for what is an increasing connection between IgE antibodies, glycosylation, and co-receptors with biologic relevance.

With IgE glycosylation likely to be a significant factor in its biology and effector function, identification of relevant patterns associated with clinical disease will be critical. Once the specific glycan patterns associated with pathology are identified and the basic biology elucidated, novel diagnostic and therapeutic therapies can be extrapolated. Glycoengineering is an exciting future prospect where in vivo generation of antibody specific glycosylation could be utilized for reduction in inflammation. Indeed, modulation of IgG and tumor glycosylation has been reported by a number of groups, highlighting the therapeutic potential of these approaches (Albert et al. 2008; Xiao et al. 2016; Pagan et al. 2018). This may be one strategy of many to target IgE glycosylation for therapeutic benefit in the futures.

Acknowledgements This work was supported by grants from the National Institutes of Health (DP2AR068272-01), and Food Allergy, Research, and Education (FARE) to RMA. We would like to apologize to all our colleagues whose important work was not cited here.

References

2010 Asthma's Impact on the Nation; Data from the CDC National Asthma Control Program. Center for Disease Control

Ackerman ME, Crispin M, Yu X, Baruah K, Boesch AW, Harvey DJ, Dugast AS, Heizen EL, Ercan A, Choi I, Streeck H, Nigrovic PA, Bailey-Kellogg C, Scanlan C, Alter G (2013a) Natural variation in Fc glycosylation of HIV-specific antibodies impacts antiviral activity. J Clin Invest 123(5):2183–2192. https://doi.org/10.1172/JCI65708

Ackerman ME, Dugast AS, McAndrew EG, Tsoukas S, Licht AF, Irvine DJ, Alter G (2013b) Enhanced phagocytic activity of HIV-specific antibodies correlates with natural production of immunoglobulins with skewed affinity for FcγR2a and FcγR2b. J Virol 87(10):5468–5476. https://doi.org/10.1128/JVI.03403-12

Albert H, Collin M, Dudziak D, Ravetch JV, Nimmerjahn F (2008) In vivo enzymatic modulation of IgG glycosylation inhibits autoimmune disease in an IgG subclass-dependent manner. Proc Natl Acad Sci U S A 105(39):15005–15009. https://doi.org/10.1073/pnas.0808248105

Anthony RM, Rutitzky LI, Urban JF Jr, Stadecker MJ, Gause WC (2007) Protective immune mechanisms in helminth infection. Nat Rev Immunol 7(12):975–987. https://doi.org/10.1038/nri2199

Anthony RM, Nimmerjahn F, Ashline DJ, Reinhold VN, Paulson JC, Ravetch JV (2008) Recapitulation of IVIG anti-inflammatory activity with a recombinant IgG Fc. Science 320 (5874):373–376

Armitage RJ, Goff LK, Beverley PC (1989) Expression and functional role of CD23 on T cells. Eur J Immunol 19(1):31–35. https://doi.org/10.1002/eji.1830190106

Arnold JN, Radcliffe CM, Wormald MR, Royle L, Harvey DJ, Crispin M, Dwek RA, Sim RB, Rudd PM (2004) The glycosylation of human serum IgD and IgE and the accessibility of identified oligomannose structures for interaction with mannan-binding lectin. J Immunol 173 (11):6831–6840

Bambouskova M, Polakovicova I, Halova I, Goel G, Draberova L, Bugajev V, Doan A, Utekal P, Gardet A, Xavier RJ, Draber P (2016) New regulatory roles of Galectin-3 in high-affinity IgE receptor signaling. Mol Cell Biol 36(9):1366–1382. https://doi.org/10.1128/MCB.00064-16

Basu M, Hakimi J, Dharm E, Kondas JA, Tsien WH, Pilson RS, Lin P, Gilfillan A, Haring P, Braswell EH et al (1993) Purification and characterization of human recombinant IgE-Fc fragments that bind to the human high affinity IgE receptor. J Biol Chem 268(18):13118–13127

Bjorklund JE, Karlsson T, Magnusson CG (1999) N-glycosylation influences epitope expression and receptor binding structures in human IgE. Mol Immunol 36(3):213–221

Bjorklund JE, Schmidt M, Magnusson CG (2000) Characterisation of recombinant human IgE-Fc fragments expressed in baculovirus-infected insect cells. Mol Immunol 37(3–4):169–177

Chang TW (2000) The pharmacological basis of anti-IgE therapy. Nat Biotechnol 18(2):157–162. https://doi.org/10.1038/72601

Cornejo-Garcia JA, Romano A, Gueant-Rodriguez RM, Oussalah A, Blanca-Lopez N, Gaeta F, Tramoy D, Josse T, Dona I, Torres MJ, Canto G, Blanca M, Gueant JL (2016) A non-synonymous polymorphism in galectin-3 lectin domain is associated with allergic reactions to beta-lactam antibiotics. Pharmacogenomics J 16(1):79–82. https://doi.org/10.1038/tpj.2015.24

Dorrington KJ, Bennich HH (1978) Structure-function relationships in human immunoglobulin E. Immunol Rev 41:3–25

Erazo A, Kutchukhidze N, Leung M, Christ AP, Urban JF Jr, Curotto de Lafaille MA, Lafaille JJ (2007) Unique maturation program of the IgE response in vivo. Immunity 26(2):191–203. https://doi.org/10.1016/j.immuni.2006.12.006

Feige MJ, Nath S, Catharino SR, Weinfurtner D, Steinbacher S, Buchner J (2009) Structure of the murine unglycosylated IgG1 Fc fragment. J Mol Biol 391(3):599–608. S0022-2836(09) 00768-2 [pii] 10.1016/j.jmb.2009.06.048

Ferrara C, Grau S, Jager C, Sondermann P, Brunker P, Waldhauer I, Hennig M, Ruf A, Rufer AC, Stihle M, Umana P, Benz J (2011) Unique carbohydrate-carbohydrate interactions are required for high affinity binding between Fc{γ}RIII and antibodies lacking core fucose. Proc Natl Acad Sci U S A 108(31):12669–74. 1108455108 [pii] 10.1073/pnas.1108455108

Fitzsimmons CM, Falcone FH, Dunne DW (2014) Helminth allergens, parasite-specific IgE, and Its protective role in human immunity. Front Immunol 5:61. https://doi.org/10.3389/fimmu.2014.00061

Frigeri LG, Zuberi RI, Liu FT (1993) Epsilon BP, a beta-galactoside-binding animal lectin, recognizes IgE receptor (Fc epsilon RI) and activates mast cells. Biochemistry 32(30):7644–7649

Gao P, Gibson PG, Baines KJ, Yang IA, Upham JW, Reynolds PN, Hodge S, James AL, Jenkins C, Peters MJ, Zhang J, Simpson JL (2015) Anti-inflammatory deficiencies in neutrophilic asthma: reduced galectin-3 and IL-1RA/IL-1β. Respir Res 16:5. https://doi.org/10.1186/s12931-014-0163-5

Garman SC, Wurzburg BA, Tarchevskaya SS, Kinet JP, Jardetzky TS (2000) Structure of the Fc fragment of human IgE bound to its high-affinity receptor FcεRIα. Nature 406(6793):259–266. https://doi.org/10.1038/35018500

Geha RS, Jabara HH, Brodeur SR (2003) The regulation of immunoglobulin E class-switch recombination. Nat Rev Immunol 3(9):721–732. https://doi.org/10.1038/nri1181

Gould HJ, Sutton BJ (2008) IgE in allergy and asthma today. Nat Rev Immunol 8(3):205–217. https://doi.org/10.1038/nri2273

Gould HJ, Sutton BJ, Beavil AJ, Beavil RL, McCloskey N, Coker HA, Fear D, Smurthwaite L (2003) The biology of IGE and the basis of allergic disease. Annu Rev Immunol 21:579–628. https://doi.org/10.1146/annurev.immunol.21.120601.141103

Gurish MF, Austen KF (2012) Developmental origin and functional specialization of mast cell subsets. Immunity 37(1):25–33. https://doi.org/10.1016/j.immuni.2012.07.003

Harris MB, Chang CC, Berton MT, Danial NN, Zhang J, Kuehner D, Ye BH, Kvatyuk M, Pandolfi PP, Cattoretti G, Dalla-Favera R, Rothman PB (1999) Transcriptional repression of Stat6-dependent interleukin-4-induced genes by BCL-6: specific regulation of iε transcription and immunoglobulin E switching. Mol Cell Bio 19:7264–7275

He JS, Meyer-Hermann M, Xiangying D, Zuan LY, Jones LA, Ramakrishna L, de Vries VC, Dolpady J, Aina H, Joseph S, Narayanan S, Subramaniam S, Puthia M, Wong G, Xiong H, Poidinger M, Urban JF, Lafaille JJ, Curotto de Lafaille MA (2013) The distinctive germinal center phase of IgE+ B lymphocytes limits their contribution to the classical memory response. J Exp Med 210(12):2755–2771. https://doi.org/10.1084/jem.20131539

He JS, Narayanan S, Subramaniam S, Ho WQ, Lafaille JJ, Curotto de Lafaille MA (2015) Biology of IgE production: IgE cell differentiation and the memory of IgE responses. Curr Top Microbiol Immunol 388:1–19. https://doi.org/10.1007/978-3-319-13725-4_1

He JS, Subramaniam S, Narang V, Srinivasan K, Saunders SP, Carbajo D, Wen-Shan T, Hidayah Hamadee N, Lum J, Lee A, Chen J, Poidinger M, Zolezzi F, Lafaille JJ, Curotto de Lafaille MA (2017) IgG1 memory B cells keep the memory of IgE responses. Nat Commun 8 (1):641. https://doi.org/10.1038/s41467-017-00723-0

Hebenstreit D, Wirnsberger G, Horejs-Hoeck J, Duschl A (2006) Signaling mechanisms, interaction partners, and target genes of STAT6. Cytokine Growth Factor Rev 17(3):173–188. https://doi.org/10.1016/j.cytogfr.2006.01.004

Helm BA, Sayers I, Padlan EA, McKendrick JE, Spivey AC (1998) Structure/function studies on IgE as a basis for the development of rational IgE antagonists. Allergy 53(45 Suppl):77–82

Helm B, Marsh P, Vercelli D, Padlan E, Gould H, Geha R (1988) The mast cell binding site on human immunoglobulin E. Nature 331(6152):180–183. https://doi.org/10.1038/331180a0

Henault J, Riggs JM, Karnell JL, Liarski VM, Li J, Shirinian L, Xu L, Casey KA, Smith MA, Khatry DB, Izhak L, Clarke L, Herbst R, Ettinger R, Petri M, Clark MR, Mustelin T, Kolbeck R, Sanjuan MA (2016) Self-reactive IgE exacerbates interferon responses associated with autoimmunity. Nat Immunol 17(2):196–203. https://doi.org/10.1038/ni.3326

Henry AJ, McDonnell JM, Ghirlando R, Sutton BJ, Gould HJ (2000) Conformation of the isolated cε3 domain of IgE and its complex with the high-affinity receptor, FcεRI. Biochemistry 39 (25):7406–7413

Holdom MD, Davies AM, Nettleship JE, Bagby SC, Dhaliwal B, Girardi E, Hunt J, Gould HJ, Beavil AJ, McDonnell JM, Owens RJ, Sutton BJ (2011) Conformational changes in IgE contribute to its uniquely slow dissociation rate from receptor FcεRI. Nat Struct Mol Biol 18 (5):571–576. https://doi.org/10.1038/nsmb.2044

Holgate ST, Church MK (1982) Control of mediator release from mast cells. Clin Allergy 12(Suppl):5–13

Holland SM, DeLeo FR, Elloumi HZ, Hsu AP, Uzel G, Brodsky N, Freeman AF, Demidowich A, Davis J, Turner ML, Anderson VL, Darnell DN, Welch PA, Kuhns DB, Frucht DM, Malech HL, Gallin JI, Kobayashi SD, Whitney AR, Voyich JM, Musser JM, Woellner C, Schaffer AA, Puck JM, Grimbacher B (2007) STAT3 mutations in the hyper-IgE syndrome. N Engl J Med 357(16):1608–1619. https://doi.org/10.1056/NEJMoa073687

Hunt J, Beavil RL, Calvert RA, Gould HJ, Sutton BJ, Beavil AJ (2005) Disulfide linkage controls the affinity and stoichiometry of IgE Fcε3-4 binding to FcεRI. J Biol Chem 280(17):16808–16814. https://doi.org/10.1074/jbc.M500965200

Jabs F, Plum M, Laursen NS, Jensen RK, Molgaard B, Miehe M, Mandolesi M, Rauber MM, Pfutzner W, Jakob T, Mobs C, Andersen GR, Spillner E (2018) Trapping IgE in a closed conformation by mimicking CD23 binding prevents and disrupts FcεRI interaction. Nat Commun 9(1):7. https://doi.org/10.1038/s41467-017-02312-7

Janeway CA, Travers P, Walport M, Shlomchik M (2001) Immunobiology. In: The immune system in health and disease, 5 edn. Garland Publishing, New York

Jankovic D, Kullberg MC, Dombrowicz D, Barbieri S, Caspar P, Wynn TA, Paul WE, Cheever AW, Kinet JP, Sher A (1997) Fc epsilonRI-deficient mice infected with *Schistosoma mansoni* mount normal Th2-type responses while displaying enhanced liver pathology. J Immunol 159:1868–1875

Kaneko Y, Nimmerjahn F, Ravetch JV (2006) Anti-inflammatory activity of immunoglobulin G resulting from Fc sialylation. Science 313(5787):670–673

Kim B, Eggel A, Tarchevskaya SS, Vogel M, Prinz H, Jardetzky TS (2012) Accelerated disassembly of IgE-receptor complexes by a disruptive macromolecular inhibitor. Nature 491(7425):613–617. https://doi.org/10.1038/nature11546

Kraft S, Kinet JP (2007) New developments in FcεRI regulation, function and inhibition. Nat Rev Immunol 7(5):365–378. https://doi.org/10.1038/nri2072

Krapp S, Mimura Y, Jefferis R, Huber R, Sondermann P (2003) Structural analysis of human IgG-Fc glycoforms reveals a correlation between glycosylation and structural integrity. J Mol Biol 325(5):979–989

Liu FT, Frigeri LG, Gritzmacher CA, Hsu DK, Robertson MW, Zuberi RI (1993) Expression and function of an IgE-binding animal lectin (εBP) in mast cells. Immunopharmacology 26(3): 187–195

Liu H, Archer NK, Dillen CA, Wang Y, Ashbaugh AG, Ortines RV, Lee SK, Kao T, Miller LS (2017) Keratinocyte-specific deletion of STAT3 promotes elevated serum IgE in response to *Staphylococcus aureus* exposure: relevance to hyper-IgE syndrome. J Immunol 198:194–208

Mandler R, Finkelman FD, Levine AD, Snapper CM (1993) IL-4 induction of IgE class switching by lipopolysaccharide-activated murine B cells occurs predominantly through sequential switching. J Immunol 150:407–418

Marichal T, Starkl P, Reber LL, Kalesnikoff J, Oettgen HC, Tsai M, Metz M, Galli SJ (2013) A beneficial role for immunoglobulin E in host defense against honeybee venom. Immunity 39 (5):963–975. https://doi.org/10.1016/j.immuni.2013.10.005

Matsumoto A, Shikata K, Takeuchi F, Kojima N, Mizuochi T (2000) Autoantibody activity of IgG rheumatoid factor increases with decreasing levels of galactosylation and sialylation. J Biochem 128(4):621–628

McCloskey N, Hunt J, Beavil RL, Jutton MR, Grundy GJ, Girardi E, Fabiane SM, Fear DJ, Conrad DH, Sutton BJ, Gould HJ (2007) Soluble CD23 monomers inhibit and oligomers stimulate IGE synthesis in human B cells. J Biol Chem 282(33):24083–24091. https://doi.org/10.1074/jbc.M703195200

Metz M, Piliponsky AM, Chen CC, Lammel V, Abrink M, Pejler G, Tsai M, Galli SJ (2006) Mast cells can enhance resistance to snake and honeybee venoms. Science 313(5786):526–530. https://doi.org/10.1126/science.1128877

Milner JD, Brenchley JM, Laurence A, Freeman AF, Hill BJ, Elias KM, Kanno Y, Spalding C, Elloumi HZ, Paulson ML, Davis J, Hsu A, Asher AI, O'Shea J, Holland SM, Paul WE, Douek DC (2008) Impaired T(H)17 cell differentiation in subjects with autosomal dominant hyper-IgE syndrome. Nature 452(7188):773–776. https://doi.org/10.1038/nature06764

Misaghi S, Senger K, Sai T, Qu Y, Sun Y, Hamidzadeh K, Nguyen A, Jin Z, Zhou M, Yan D, Lin WY, Lin Z, Lorenzo MN, Sebrell A, Ding J, Xu M, Caplazi P, Austin CD, Balazs M, Roose-Girma M, DeForge L, Warming S, Lee WP, Dixit VM, Zarrin AA (2013) Polyclonal hyper-IgE mouse model reveals mechanistic insights into antibody class switch recombination. Proc Natl Acad Sci U S A 110(39):15770–15775. https://doi.org/10.1073/pnas.1221661110

Miyawaki S, Ritchie RF (1973) Nucleolar antigen specfic for antinucleolar antibody in the sera of patients with rheumatologic disease. Arthritis Rheum 16:726–736

Mogensen TH (2016) Primary immunodeficiencies with elevated IgE. Int Rev Immunol 35(1):39–56. https://doi.org/10.3109/08830185.2015.1027820

Mukai K, Tsai M, Starkl P, Marichal T, Galli SJ (2016) IgE and mast cells in host defense against parasites and venoms. Semin Immunopathol 38(5):581–603. https://doi.org/10.1007/s00281-016-0565-1

Nettleton MY, Kochan JP (1995) Role of glycosylation sites in the IgE Fc molecule. Int Arch Allergy Immunol 107(1–3):328–329

Nieminen P, Morgan NV, Fenwick AL, Parmanen S, Veistinen L, Mikkola ML, van der Spek PJ, Giraud A, Judd L, Arte S, Brueton LA, Wall SA, Mathijssen IM, Maher ER, Wilkie AO, Kreiborg S, Thesleff I (2011) Inactivation of IL11 signaling causes craniosynostosis, delayed tooth eruption, and supernumerary teeth. Am J Hum Genet 89(1):67–81. https://doi.org/10.1016/j.ajhg.2011.05.024

Niki T, Tsutsui S, Hirose S, Aradono S, Sugimoto Y, Takeshita K, Nishi N, Hirashima M (2009) Galectin-9 is a high affinity IgE-binding lectin with anti-allergic effect by blocking IgE-antigen complex formation. J Biol Chem 284(47):32344–32352. https://doi.org/10.1074/jbc.M109.035196

Pagan JD, Kitaoka M, Anthony RM (2018) Engineered sialylation of pathogenic antibodies in vivo attenuates autoimmune disease. Cell. https://doi.org/10.1016/j.cell.2017.11.041

Palaniyandi S, Tomei E, Li Z, Conrad DH, Zhu X (2011) CD23-dependent transcytosis of IgE and immune complex across the polarized human respiratory epithelial cells. J Immunol 186(6):3484–3496. https://doi.org/10.4049/jimmunol.1002146

Palm NW, Rosenstein RK, Yu S, Schenten DD, Florsheim E, Medzhitov R (2013) Bee venom phospholipase A2 induces a primary type 2 response that is dependent on the receptor ST2 and confers protective immunity. Immunity 39(5):976–985. https://doi.org/10.1016/j.immuni.2013.10.006

Pawankar R, Canonica GW, Holgate S, Lockey RF (2011). WAO white book on allergy 2011–2012: executive summary. https://www.worldallergy.org/UserFiles/file/WAO-White-Book-on-Allergy_web.pdf

Pincetic A, Bournazos S, DiLillo DJ, Maamary J, Wang TT, Dahan R, Fiebiger BM, Ravetch JV (2014) Type I and type II Fc receptors regulate innate and adaptive immunity. Nat Immunol 15(8):707–716. https://doi.org/10.1038/ni.2939

Plomp R, Hensbergen PJ, Rombouts Y, Zauner G, Dragan I, Koeleman CA, Deelder AM, Wuhrer M (2013) Site-specific N-glycosylation analysis of human immunoglobulin E. J Proteome Res. https://doi.org/10.1021/pr400714w

Reinhardt RL, Liang HE, Locksley RM (2009) Cytokine-secreting follicular T cells shape the antibody repertoire. Nat Immunol 10(4):385–393. https://doi.org/10.1038/ni.1715

Riccio AM, Mauri P, De Ferrari L, Rossi R, Di Silvestre D, Benazzi L, Chiappori A, Dal Negro RW, Micheletto C, Canonica GW (2017) Galectin-3: an early predictive biomarker of modulation of airway remodeling in patients with severe asthma treated with omalizumab for 36 months. Clin Transl Allergy 7:6. https://doi.org/10.1186/s13601-017-0143-1

Rieber EP, Rank G, Kohler I, Krauss S (1993) Membrane expression of Fc ε RII/CD23 and release of soluble CD23 by follicular dendritic cells. Adv Exp Med Biol 329:393–398

Ronnblom L, Alm GV (2001) A pivotal role for the natural interferon α-producing cells (plasmacytoid dendritic cells) in the pathogenesis of lupus. J Exp Med 194:F59–F63

Sayers I, Cain SA, Swan JR, Pickett MA, Watt PJ, Holgate ST, Padlan EA, Schuck P, Helm BA (1998) Amino acid residues that influence FcεRI-mediated effector functions of human immunoglobulin E. Biochemistry 37(46):16152–16164. https://doi.org/10.1021/bi981456k

Scherer HU, van der Woude D, Ioan-Facsinay A, el Bannoudi H, Trouw LA, Wang J, Haupl T, Burmester GR, Deelder AM, Huizinga TW, Wuhrer M, Toes RE (2010) Glycan profiling of anti-citrullinated protein antibodies isolated from human serum and synovial fluid. Arthritis Rheum 62(6):1620–1629. https://doi.org/10.1002/art.27414

Shade KT, Platzer B, Washburn N, Mani V, Bartsch YC, Conroy M, Pagan JD, Bosques C, Mempel TR, Fiebiger E, Anthony RM (2015) A single glycan on IgE is indispensable for initiation of anaphylaxis. J Exp Med 212(4):457–467. https://doi.org/10.1084/jem.20142182

Shields RL, Lai J, Keck R, O'Connell LY, Hong K, Meng YG, Weikert SH, Presta LG (2002) Lack of fucose on human IgG1N-linked oligosaccharide improves binding to human Fcγ RIII and antibody-dependent cellular toxicity. J Biol Chem 277(30):26733–26740

Siegel AM, Heimall J, Freeman AF, Hsu AP, Brittain E, Brenchley JM, Douek DC, Fahle GH, Cohen JI, Holland SM, Milner JD (2011) A critical role for STAT3 transcription factor signaling in the development and maintenance of human T cell memory. Immunity 35(5):806–818. https://doi.org/10.1016/j.immuni.2011.09.016

Sondermann P, Huber R, Oosthuizen V, Jacob U (2000) The 3.2-a crystal structure of the human IgG1 Fc fragment-FcγRIII complex. Nature 406(6793):267–273. https://doi.org/10.1038/35018508

Sondermann P, Pincetic A, Maamary J, Lammens K, Ravetch JV (2013) General mechanism for modulating immunoglobulin effector function. Proc Natl Acad Sci U S A. https://doi.org/10.1073/pnas.1307864110

Sowerwine KJ, Holland SM, Freeman AF (2012) Hyper-IgE syndrome update. Ann N Y Acad Sci 1250:25–32. https://doi.org/10.1111/j.1749-6632.2011.06387.x

van de Geijn FE, Wuhrer M, Selman MH, Willemsen SP, de Man YA, Deelder AM, Hazes JM, Dolhain RJ (2009) Immunoglobulin G galactosylation and sialylation are associated with pregnancy-induced improvement of rheumatoid arthritis and the postpartum flare: results from a large prospective cohort study. Arthritis Res Ther 11(6):R193. ar2892 [pii] 10.1186/ar2892

Vercelli D, Helm B, Marsh P, Padlan E, Geha RS, Gould H (1989) The B-cell binding site on human immunoglobulin E. Nature 338(6217):649–651. https://doi.org/10.1038/338649a0

Vieira P, Rajewsky K (1988) The half-lives of serum immunoglobulins in adult mice. Eur J Immunol 18(2):313–316. https://doi.org/10.1002/eji.1830180221

Wan T, Beavil RL, Fabiane SM, Beavil AJ, Sohi MK, Keown M, Young RJ, Henry AJ, Owens RJ, Gould HJ, Sutton BJ (2002) The crystal structure of IgE Fc reveals an asymmetrically bent conformation. Nat Immunol 3(7):681–686. https://doi.org/10.1038/ni811

Wesemann DR, Magee JM, Boboila C, Calado DP, Gallagher MP, Portuguese AJ, Manis JP, Zhou X, Recher M, Rajewsky K, Notarangelo LD, Alt FW (2011) Immature B cells preferentially switch to IgE with increased direct Sμ to Sε recombination. J Exp Med 208(13):2733–2746. https://doi.org/10.1084/jem.20111155

Wesemann DR, Portuguese AJ, Magee JM, Gallagher MP, Zhou X, Panchakshari RA, Alt FW (2012) Reprogramming IgH isotype-switched B cells to functional-grade induced pluripotent stem cells. Proc Natl Acad Sci U S A 109(34):13745–13750. https://doi.org/10.1073/pnas.1210286109

Wu G, Hitchen PG, Panico M, North SJ, Barbouche MR, Binet D, Morris HR, Dell A, Haslam SM (2016) Glycoproteomic studies of IgE from a novel hyper IgE syndrome linked to PGM3 mutation. Glycoconj J 33(3):447–456. https://doi.org/10.1007/s10719-015-9638-y

Wuhrer M, Stam JC, van de Geijn FE, Koeleman CA, Verrips CT, Dolhain RJ, Hokke CH, Deelder AM (2007) Glycosylation profiling of immunoglobulin G (IgG) subclasses from human serum. Proteomics 7(22):4070–4081. https://doi.org/10.1002/pmic.200700289

Wurzburg BA, Garman SC, Jardetzky TS (2000) Structure of the human IgE-Fc C epsilon 3-C epsilon 4 reveals conformational flexibility in the antibody effector domains. Immunity 13(3): 375–385

Xiao H, Woods EC, Vukojicic P, Bertozzi CR (2016) Precision glycocalyx editing as a strategy for cancer immunotherapy. Proc Natl Acad Sci U S A 113(37):10304–10309. https://doi.org/10. 1073/pnas.1608069113

Yang Z, Sullivan BM, Allen CD (2012) Fluorescent in vivo detection reveals that IgE(+) B cells are restrained by an intrinsic cell fate predisposition. Immunity 36(5):857–872. https://doi.org/ 10.1016/j.immuni.2012.02.009

Young RJ, Owens RJ, Mackay GA, Chan CM, Shi J, Hide M, Francis DM, Henry AJ, Sutton BJ, Gould HJ (1995) Secretion of recombinant human IgE-Fc by mammalian cells and biological activity of glycosylation site mutants. Protein Eng 8(2):193–199

Yu LC, Montagnac G, Yang PC, Conrad DH, Benmerah A, Perdue MH (2003) Intestinal epithelial CD23 mediates enhanced antigen transport in allergy: evidence for novel splice forms. Am J Physiol Gastrointest Liver Physiol 285(1):G223–G234. https://doi.org/10.1152/ajpgi.00445. 2002

Zuberi RI, Frigeri LG, Liu FT (1994) Activation of rat basophilic leukemia cells by ϵBP, an IgE-binding endogenous lectin. Cell Immunol 156(1):1–12

Immune Complex Vaccination

Yu-mei Wen and Yan Shi

Contents

Y. Wen (✉)
Key Laboratory of Molecular Virology, Shanghai Medical College,
School of Basic Medical Sciences, Fudan University, Shanghai, China
e-mail: ymwen@shmu.edu.cn

Shanghai Medical College, Fudan University, Rm 401, Fuxing Bldg,
131 Yi Xue Yuan Rd, Shanghai 200032, China

Y. Shi
Department of Basic Medical Sciences, Center for Life Sciences,
Institute of Immunology, Tsinghua University, Beijing, China
e-mail: yanshiemail@mail.tsinghua.edu.cn

Department of Microbiology, Immunology & Infectious Diseases and Snyder Institute
for Chronic Diseases, University of Calgary, Calgary, AB, Canada

D301 Medical Sciences Bldg, Tsinghua University, Beijing 00084, China

Current Topics in Microbiology and Immunology (2019) 423: 95–118
https://doi.org/10.1007/82_2019_153
© Springer Nature Switzerland AG 2019
Published online: 22 February 2019

Abstract Antibody/antigen binding results in immune complexes (IC) that have a variety of regulatory functions. One important feature is the enhanced host immune activation against antigen contained in the complex. ICs play important roles at several critical steps that lead to B and T cell activation, including antigen targeting/retention, facilitated antigen uptake, antigen presenting cell activation and proper balancing of positive and negative stimulatory signals. In both poultry industry and clinical health care, ICs have been used as preventive and therapeutic vaccines. With our deepening understanding of antibody biology, particularly in light of new revelations of regulatory functions of Fc receptors, mechanistically more precise engineering has spearheaded tailored use of this tool for infection control and cancer therapy. IC-based treatment and prophylaxis have been tested to different extents in HBV, HIV and influenza viral infection control and are actively examined as an alternative treatment for several forms of tumor. As a part of this book series, this chapter aims to discuss the mechanistic aspects of IC signaling and their impact on immune cells. We give samples how this old technology has been used by practitioners over the last several decades and suggest potential paths for future development of IC-based immune therapy.

1 Introduction

Translational applications of research on immune complexes (IC) have resulted in the development of immune complex vaccines. In contrast to pathological outcomes induced by IC deposition, vaccines in various forms of ICs have led to facilitated antigen uptake by antigen presenting cells (APC), modified processing, and enhanced humoral and cellular immune responses in disease therapies and prophylaxis. In the poultry industry, IC vaccines have been highly successful in preventing viral outbreaks in newborn chickens. In clinical settings, human IC vaccines induce higher antibody titers with concomitant broader coverage. In addition to promoting effective antibodies, IC vaccines are also capable of mediating cellular immune responses that target persistently infected cells. This feature is desired in the development of therapeutic vaccines against chronical viral infections, such as HIV and Hepatitis viruses. With our deepening understanding of Fc subtypes and the divergent functions of Fcγ receptors, more tailored IC preparations designed to fully utilize the specific antibody/FcγR pairing have opened up a door to an even more promising future. Here, we provide a summary of the current experimental and clinical investigations into IC vaccines and a discussion on the mechanisms of IC's immune-enhancing effects.

Vaccination is one of the most effective public health measures of controlling infectious diseases, lowering disease burden and increasing life expectancy on a demographic scale. The basic goal of preventive vaccines is to elicit host immune responses against microbial infections, which includes facilitated recall responses of specific antibodies and antigen-specific T cells in the case of real infection challenge by the microbes bearing the same antigen. Mechanistically, the magnitude and the quality of the adaptive immune responses largely rely on the native and more ubiquitous innate immune activation, and the use of adjuvants is the most established method to trigger the innate immunity. To enhance the immunogenicity of vaccines, a number of adjuvants have been developed, but only alum and few others have been licensed for use. Even under the limited selection, the use of adjuvants has led to development of several most successful vaccines in the history targeting DTP (Diphtheria–Tetanus–Pertussis combination), HBV, influenza and pneumococcal pneumonia (Kool et al. 2012; Wen and Shi 2016). With the emerging prevalence of drug-resistant microbes, vaccination has become an even more important tool for infection control. In recent years, together with the use of prophylactic immunization, therapeutic vaccines and immunotherapies are also under rapid development, targeting persistent infections and tumors. In comparison with the anti-infectious purposes, the latter is still in its early stage exploration but is expected to hold great promise. Regardless the purpose, in the long history of vaccine development, the aim of researchers and manufacturers has always been to improve vaccine efficacies and to decrease its side effects. Among the tools at hand, immune complexes are one of them.

In vaccine preparations about a century ago, antibodies were added to antigens such as diphtheria toxin to decrease its toxicity (Copeman et al. 1922). For the same amount of antigen, enhanced immunity to antigen in complex with antibody was first reported by Terres et al. They found that when bovine serum albumin was mixed with its specific antibody the resulting complex induced a stronger antibody response in mice, compared to those immunized with antigen alone, or complexed to a non-relevant antibody (Terres and Wolins 1959, 1961). Using the same amount of antigen, ICs were much more effective than alum-precipitated antigen (Morrison and Terres 1966). After three decades, Berzofsky et al. used peptides from HIV gp120 to rejuvenate CD4 cells in HIV carriers and found that addition of antibodies that recognized the peptides substantially increased the proliferation index of the CD4 T cells in the patients (Berzofsky et al. 1988). Around the same time, Celis and Chang et al. performed a series of in vitro human HBsAg-specific T cells and HBsAg co-culture experiments. They showed that monoclonal antibodies to HBsAg of the IgG subclass increased the amount of HBsAg captured and internalized by APCs in vitro. In addition, mouse monoclonal antibodies when presented with HBsAg as IC enhanced the proliferation of T cell clones specific to HBsAg by about two logs and increased the specific production of IFN-γ (Celis et al. 1984, 1987; Celis and Chang 1984). Similarly, Randall et al. reported that by using an SMAA (solid matrix antibody-antigen complex) approach, antigen-antibody complex attached to Staphylococcus aureus Cowan I strain via the Fc fragment induced effective humoral and cytotoxic T cell responses to simian virus 5 protein in a persistently infected mouse model (Randall and Young 1988). In a follow-up report, specific CD8 T cells were found responsible for the clearance of the persistent virus (Randall and Young 1991).

Those advancements gradually established that antigen-antibody ICs can significantly increase the immunogenicity of antigens. However, to a large extent, those practices were empirical in nature. In recent years, the development of Fc receptor biology has completely revamped the research on this "old" weapon, paving the way for much broader and more precise use of ICs in the control of acute and chronic infections as well as several forms of tumor. As antibody-based therapies (without explicit intension to induce ICs) are covered in other reviews, this chapter will focus on the general mechanisms and clinical/industrial applications of ICs in disease control.

2 How ICs Enhance Immune Responses

2.1 Fcγ Receptors in IC/Antigen Uptake, Processing and Presentation

FcγRs are quintessential to our understanding of IC functions and are therefore discussed here first. In the middle of the last century, reports surfaced that indicated the possible presence of a moiety on the immune cell membrane that was essential to IC-mediated immune effects. The Fc portion of antibodies seemed to exert regulatory roles in addition to specificity determinants in Fabs (Berken and Benacerraf 1966; Boyden and Sorkin 1960). In the later years, several key reports described the presence of Fc receptors on the surface of cells of the immune system (Ravetch and Kinet 1991). By the 1980s, most common forms of FcγRs were identified, except for mouse FcγRIV which was cloned in 2005 (Nimmerjahn et al. 2005). In mice, IgG receptors are made of FcγRI, IIB, III and IV. The human counterparts include FcγRIA, FcγRIIA, FcγRIIB. FcγRIIC, FcγRIIIA and FcγRIIIB. Among them, signaling mechanism of human FcγRIIIB, a GPI-anchored protein, remains elusive although it is known to induce Ca2+ flux in neutrophils (Marois et al. 2011). Both FcγRIIBs contain an intracellular ITIM (immunoreceptor tyrosine-based inhibitory motif) signaling domain and are considered inhibitory and the sole antagonist in the type I FcγR family. All other FcγRs transduce activating signal via an ITAM (immunoreceptor tyrosine-based activation motif) present either in the associated common γ chain or intrinsic to its intracellular sequence. In mice, IgG1, IgG2a (IgG2c in C57BL/6), IgG2b, and IgG3, and in human, IgG1–4 are their respective ligands. Affinity wise, all FcγRs are silent in the absence of cross-linking, in other words, incapable to signal without higher orders formed in ICs, except for FcγIR. FcγIR has an extra immunoglobulin domain that permits the highest affinity and binding of IgG monomer without involving receptor cross-linking. The rest of FcγRs displays different affinities to different subtypes IgGs. As each receptor/ligand pair affinity varies, the FcγRs are exposed to multiple IgG subtypes simultaneously, FcγR signaling on a given cell type can be difficult to predict. In addition to the affinity differences, cell type/activation stage-specific expression, ITAM versus ITIM-based signaling and competition from type II FcγRs tuned by the different glycosylation states of Fc introduce several variables into FcγR regulation, creating the mesmerizing complexity. Up to this day, an important task is to precisely map the affinity and in vivo pairing of subtypes of Fc and their FcRs (Boesch et al. 2014). These complex interactions are expertly covered by other reviews (Bournazos et al. 2015; Lux et al. 2013). Overall, we are just beginning to understand how ICs interact with different FcRs (Bruhns 2012; Lux et al. 2013), and a great deal of work is still needed before the concept of IgG/FcR pairing can be fully utilized in the clinics.

2.2 Other Fcγ Receptors

In addition to type I FcγRs, type II FcγRs (DC-SIGN and CD23) are lectin-based Fc receptors that are sensitive to the glycosylation state of Fc. A prominent example is the glycosylation extended from a glycan core at N297. A number of sugar moieties can be attached to this structure, such as fucose, galactose and sialic acid. One way this pattern of glycosylation can modify the FcγR binding is to introduce a greater flexibility of the antibody heavy chain. For instance, the presence of sialic acid allows open conformation of the heavy chain that leads to its preferential binding to type II FcγRs. This switch in binding affinity therefore is immune-regulatory and is in general considered inhibitory (Pincetic et al. 2014). Interestingly, at least in one model, where OVA was targeted in vivo to DEC205 via an antibody without CD40 signal, IgGs produced were highly sialylated due to enhanced activity of sialyl-transferase in the plasma cells (Oefner et al. 2012). For now, the research on the signaling mechanism of type II FcγR in the context of IgG binding has just started, for instance, CD23 ligation induces FcγRIIB expression and participates in the affinity maturation of BCRs (Wang et al. 2015), although a lot of work remains.

A nomenclature-related structure, neonatal FcR (FcRn) is a MHC class I-related protein associated with β2 m. This endosomal protein binds to IgG in low pH environment (pH < 6.5) and plays a role of IgG transporter in epithelial/endothelial cells. A chimeric antibody with Fc mutations that disrupts FcRn binding without affecting FcγR affinity shows reduced antigen presentation to CD4 T cells from the bound OVA (Qiao et al. 2008). A Fc mutant with enhanced binding to FcRn increases MHC class II antigen presentation, apparently via efficient lysosome targeting (Mi et al. 2008). In addition, FcRn can be used as a tool to target antigens to mucosal sites (Gosselin et al. 2009; Hioe et al. 2009), as exemplified by the delivery of live simian immunodeficiency virus (SIV) vaccine to cervical epithelium in rhesus monkey (Li et al. 2014).

2.3 Antigen Presentation

Vaccines are delivered to antigen presenting cells via internalization. The endosomal maturation leads to the degradation of engulfed antigens, which are typically loaded on the MHC class II molecules in a subset of endolysosomal vesicles called MHC class II compartment. In cross-presentation, engulfed antigens also can be delivered to MHC class I via several yet to be completely resolved pathways (Burgdorf et al. 2007; Joffre et al. 2012; Lizee et al. 2003). Cross-presentation was initially discovered using antigens coated to latex beads or as cell-associated antigens (Bevan 1976; Rock et al. 1990). It was found that antigens contained within phagocytic targets can induce CD8 T cell activation. Although this feature is typically associated with phagocytosis of solid structures, the process is subject to additional regulations. The facilitating effects of ICs were found in early attempts of antibody treatment of tumors. EG7 cells (CD4-expressing EL4 tumor line) inoculated into the host were killed by co-injection of anti-CD4 antibody. This cytolysis was dependent on CD8 T cells and the common Fc receptor γ chain (Vasovic et al. 1997). This suggested that antibody binding "sensitized" the tumor cells for immune eradication. In a later transgenic model for type I (autoimmune) diabetes, whereby a membrane-bound OVA was driven by RIP (rat insulin promoter), injection of OVA-specific CD8 T cells did not have any overt effect. However, if in the process OVA-specific IgG antibody was co-administered, the mice developed severe type I diabetes (Harbers et al. 2007). The result indicated that the antibody was needed for a robust CD8 T cell activation. As expected, the presence of FcγR was required for this facilitating effect. The enhancement of antigen presentation by ICs appears to operate at two levels. Measured by antigen uptake, the presence of ICs/FcγRs appears to increase the efficacy by two to three logs (Amigorena and Bonnerot 1999; Schuurhuis et al. 2002). However, if the effect was measured from the degree of T cell activation, the magnitude is amplified by 4–5 logs (Regnault et al. 1999). This seems to indicate that ICs/FcγR interaction can facilitate T cell activation beyond antigen uptake by APCs. Because FcR common γ chain deficiency leads to FcγR surface level reduction, an ITAM sequence mutated version (NOTAM) was created which permits FcγR expression similar to the wild type. IC uptake was restored in the NOTAM mice. In one report, IC-associated antigen cross-presentation was lost (Boross et al. 2014). However, a recent paper found that antibodies fused with antigen targeting FcγRIV and FcγRIIB/III showed no or minimal dependence on the ITAM signaling (Lehmann et al. 2017). Therefore intracellular signaling emanated from the ITAM sequence is essential for cross-presentation at least in some settings, but in other cases, such as active binding by antibodies specific for FcγRs (rather than FcR/Fc binding), the ITAM sequence may not be essential. Although most DCs can cross-present antigens in vitro, there is evidence that in vivo, CD8+ or CD103 + DCs are the main cell types involved in cross-presentation in mice. OVA-conjugated to an antibody targeting DNGR1 (a c-type lectin receptor) expressed by these cells elicited strong response against OVA-bearing B16 tumor (Sancho et al. 2008). However, whether these cells are particularly sensitive to ICs is not known. It has been reported that CD8+ DCs mediated cross-presentation without help from FcγRs, while antigen delivered in the form of ICs to FcγR was critical for CD8− DC antigen presentation to CD8+ T cells (den Haan and Bevan 2002).

For MHC class II antigen presentation, exogenous soluble antigens are engulfed via several endocytic mechanisms, such as clathrin-mediated and caveolin (lipid rafts)-mediated endocytosis. In smaller scale, these antigens can be taken up via more subtle pinocytosis or membrane ruffles. Soluble antigen endocytosis is enhanced by receptor activities, i.e., mannose, C-type lectin and cytokine receptors (Cendrowski et al. 2016). FcγR-mediated endocytosis is highly efficient and appears to enhance both MHC class II antigen presentation as well as cross-presentation to CD8+ T cells, in contrast to, i.e., the sole facilitating effects for CD4 T cell activation by mannose receptor (Berlyn et al. 2001). A mutation in the ITAM sequence that blocks Syk binding reduced the antigen delivery to the lysosome. Syk deficiency also dissociated the colocalization of DM molecule (critical for MHC class II peptide exchange from invariant chain-derived CLIP sequence to bona fide epitope sequences) with class II molecules (Le Roux et al. 2007), reducing the peptide loading efficiency. Interestingly, while both DCs and macrophages express MHC class II molecules and ICs can also efficiently target macrophages, only DCs can present antigens to cognate CD4 T cells (de Jong et al. 2006). This feature may be to a large extent due to the intracellular antigen targeting in DCs.

B cells, as a group of APCs that do not usually express activating FcγRs, cannot be activated by ICs directly. However, B cell activation can be enhanced by FcγRIIB-mediated antigen retention. Lymph node follicular DCs (FDCs) express FcγRIIB (Kosco et al. 1989; Szakal et al. 1988a, b). In vivo, the long extensions of FDCs are often coated with ICs in a FcγRIIB-dependent manner, a mechanism that avoids clearance. This provides a steady source of antigens for B cells. In addition, FcγRIIB-mediated internalization can prolong antigen presentation by "regurgitation." Large amounts of ICs can be trapped by macrophages in the subcapsular cavities. These ICs can be transferred to FDCs for FcγRIIB-based internalization. In this case, ICs are not routed into the degradative pathway. Instead, the complexes are retained inside FDCs and may reappear on the cell surface and made available to B cells (Bergtold et al. 2005; Heesters et al. 2013). This process significantly extends the duration of antigen availability and alters lymphocyte activation kinetics. This process is involved in BCR hypermutagenesis to give rise to high affinity antibodies (Wu et al. 2008).

2.4 Intracellular Targeting

IC-facilitated antigen presentation simultaneously alters intracellular targeting. This is a part of the mechanistic insight how these complexes can both qualitatively and quantitatively impact T and B cell activation. Despite the evidence that FcR common γ chain ITAM signaling is not essential in all cases (Lehmann et al. 2017), some studies implicating FcγR signaling in regulating antigen processing come from the fact that Syk deficiency blocks IC-mediate immune activation, yet Syk itself is not absolutely essential for IC antigen uptake (Boross et al. 2014). Regrettably, this finding has not led to sufficient follow up at cellular and organismic levels. IC-mediated cross-presentation appears to require TAP and is sensitive to proteasome inhibition (Regnault et al. 1999), suggesting that FcγR signaling may lead to antigen transport from endosome to cytosol or ER-phagosome fusion-based

MHC class I antigen presentation (Joffre et al. 2012). How ICs mediate these events are completely unknown. In some studies, ICs appear to retain antigen in the early endocytic vesicles (Chatterjee et al. 2012; Cohn et al. 2013), avoiding the speedy endosomal maturation that exposes antigens to the harsh acidification accompanied by the staged chain activation of vacuolar cathepsins. In this process, Cathepsin S, a neutral pH protease, takes up the bulk of peptide generation (Hari et al. 2015), which favors the production of epitope peptides. According to recent studies, the delayed antigen degradation in DCs, in comparison with macrophages and neutrophils, may be a critical feature that leads to the exceedingly strong antigen presentation by DCs (Joffre et al. 2012; Savina et al. 2006). How ICs and FcγR activation amplify this feature is not known. For MHC class II antigen presentation, ICs can help target antigens into the endolysosomal vesicles that give rise to the MHC class II compartment. Viral antigen rabies G, free or in complex of ICs, could enter Rab5+ vesicles (early endosomes). However, IC-associated rabies G then appeared in Rab9+ late endosomes while free antigen is seen colocalized with Rab11+ recycling endosome (St Pierre et al. 2011). This effect can explain the more efficient class II antigen presentation and may be not contradictory to the "shallow targeting" observed for class I cross-presentation. As the overall effect of ICs is to increase antigenic epitope availability for both pathways, IC-mediated antigen targeting may show subtle changes per cell types and antigen/FcR subtypes involved, collectively reducing the waste of antigens in the endocytic maturation process.

2.5 APC Regulation

In an early study, it was found that bone marrow-derived DCs (BMDCs) loaded with OVA/OVA-specific antibody complex induced antigen-specific humoral and CD4 and CD8 cellular responses in mice. Although total IgG was not affected by immunization, specific anti-OVA IgG responses were significantly enhanced after immunization with OVA/IC–loaded BMDCs. This immunization was able to suppress a tumor bearing the same antigen (Rafiq et al. 2002). Importantly, in this experiment, DC-specific deficiency of FcγRs, TAP, β2 m or MHC class II eliminated the tumor immunity, suggesting that ICs delivered to DCs alone is sufficient to include both humoral and cellular immunity. In accordance with this observation, ICs were later reported to empower CD8+ T cells via dual effects. First, OVA IC complex indeed increased the antigen uptake by DCs compared to OVA plus an control antibody. ICs alone also triggered IL-12 expression, suggesting a simultaneous cell activation. The specific CD8 response against the OVA epitope induced by the IC could not be replaced by OVA and LPS, pointing to IC's unique ability to prime CTL activation (Schuurhuis et al. 2002). Furthermore, ICs were shown to reprogram CD8 T cells. By using epitopes from influenza virus, Leon et al. studied ICs effects on memory CD8 T cells in mice and showed although prolonged Ag presentation did not alter the number of memory CD8 T cells, ICs were essential for programming the capacity of these cells to proliferate, produce cytokines and protect the host after secondary challenge. Importantly, prolonged Ag presentation by DCs was dependent on virus-specific, isotype-switched antibodies (Abs) that facilitated the capture and cross-presentation of viral antigens by FcγR-expressing DCs (Leon et al. 2014).

From the prospective of signaling, FcγR-mediated APC activation follows a typical immune tyrosine-based cascade common to most immune cells. The receptor binding triggers the recruitment of Syk to the phosphorylated ITAM, followed by activation of PI3Ks, PLCs, MAPKs and NFκb (Mocsai et al. 2010). In addition to organizing cytoskeleton for phagocytosis, these canonical immune activation events upregulate CD40, CD86, IL-6, IL-13 and IL-2 (Boross et al. 2014; Matsubara et al. 2006; Perreau et al. 2008). FcγR binding by ICs also sends a maturation signal that initiates the migration of DCs from the periphery to draining lymph nodes (Clatworthy et al. 2014). It has been suggested that the internalized ICs can activate intracellular TRIM21 (a non-typical Fc receptor), which leads an independent signaling chain in K63-specific Ubc13-mediated ubiquitination event. This event triggers NFκb, AP-1 and IRF pathways for synergistic activation of APCs (McEwan et al. 2013).

Depending on the setup, the FcγR signaling can be inhibitory. IVIG, the clinical application of purified whole blood immunoglobulins, binding to FcγRIII blocks macrophage activation in response to IFN-γ (Park-Min et al. 2007). In contrast to the belief that formation of ICs during chronic infection leads to inflammation, it was recently reported that in LCMV clone 13 long-term infection, ICs formed during the infection blocked the T and B cell depletion by specific antibodies and DC activation by anti-CD40 antibody (Wieland et al. 2015; Yamada et al. 2015). This inhibitory effect was dependent on the CD4 T cell-dependent antibody production.

3 Experimental and Clinical IC Vaccines

3.1 IC Vaccines in Poultry Industry

Preventive IC vaccine was first tested in poultry breeding to control infectious bursal disease (IBD), a viral infection targeting bursa of Fabricius and killing developing B cells. IBD is one of the economically most important diseases that affects commercially produced chickens worldwide. The obstacle of using conventional live IBDV vaccines was the high levels of maternal antibodies interfering with the efficacy of vaccines in chicks (Naqi et al. 1983). To overcome this obstacle, an IC vaccine was developed by mixing IBDV strain 2512 with bursal disease antibodies (BDA). One-day-old chicklings were administered IBDV-BDA, which induced active immunity and protection against a standard IBDV challenge (Haddad et al. 1997). Later in a field trial, 40,000 broiler eggs at 18 days of embryonation and 40,000 one-day-old chicks were each split into two groups. IC Vaccine (Cevac® Transmune) was either administered by in ovo, or by subcutaneous route. A highly virulent IBDV strain was used for challenge. A marked protection was reached by the IC vaccine (Iván et al. 2005). Most remarkable was the low level of bursal and splenic B cell depletion in those vaccinated with IBDV–ICs (Jeurissen et al. 1998). Furthermore, in ovo inoculation with the IBDV–IC vaccine induced more germinal centers in the spleen, and larger amounts of IBDV were deposited on splenic and bursal FDCs. It was concluded that not only in ovo IC vaccination was safe to the embryo and kept the hatchability as expected, but also a full protection against IBD was demonstrated for the broilers' lifespan. Although there are a number of IBD vaccines under development (Müller et al. 2012), IBDV–ICs have been in active use by chicken breeders in several countries. Recently, recombinant neutralizing antibodies have been developed to replace BDA previously used for IC vaccines, and the second generation of recombinant antibody-based experimental IBDV-IC vaccine is undergoing testing (Ignjatovic et al. 2006).

IC applications in the prevention of Newcastle disease virus (NDV, a flu-like infection with high death rates) have also been equally successful. Maternal IgY antibodies can protect the chicks for a short period, however, the gap of vulnerability thereafter is a window for NDV infection before the full-scale immunity is developed in more mature birds. Injection of the IgY right after hatching extends the protection. Whether this protection is completely dependent on IC formation is not clear. Commercially, NDV ICs have been produced by mixing antisera from immune chickens with the viral particles. This IC provided complete protection in broiler chickens (Pokric et al. 1993). A later report showed that in ovo application of the IC vaccine in maternal antibody–positive chickens, the birds were protected from clinical disease against three highly virulent strains of NDV (Kapczynski et al. 2013). In addition, IC vaccines for infectious anemia disease virus (CAV) in chickens are also under development (Karel A. Schat et al. 2011). In duck HBV vaccination test, one-day-old ducklings were inoculated with duck hepatitis B virus (DHBV), an infection that is persistent and somewhat mimics the human disease. They were then vaccinated with an DHBsAg IC linked to SMAA. 70 and 50% of treated ducks were cleared of viremia and antigenemia after three injections (Wen et al. 1994). This study prompted the attempts to treat persistent human HBV infections with ICs discussed later.

3.2 IC Vaccination for Influenza Virus Infection

Influenza virus belongs to the orthomyxoviridae, with its genome consisting of eight segmented RNAs that are prone to mutations and reassortments, leading to emergence of new viral strains. Due to the lack of protective antibodies to the emerging strains in the population, numerous deaths and millions of hospitalization following each outbreak are currently difficult to control. Each year, World Health

Organization collects new isolates worldwide for analysis to best predict impending danger and to prepare vaccines for all countries. It is desirable to develop a broadly protective flu vaccine which can induce immune responses against a number of influenza strains.

Recently, in a study of seasonal trivalent influenza vaccine (TIV) immunization in healthy adults, it was found that the abundance of sialylated Fc (sFc) on anti-HA (hemagglutinin) IgGs produced during the early plasmablast response correlated with vaccine efficacy. The mechanism of this enhanced antibody response involved co-engagement of CD23 by sialylated Fc domains. Mechanistically, sFc engagement of CD23 induced the inhibitory FcγRIIB expressing, setting up a high threshold for selecting high affinity BCRs (Wang et al. 2015). This observation was further extended by constructing ICs with 2014–15 TIV and sialylated Fc anti-HA IgGs that were used to immunize mice. When the sera of IC vs. HA only immunized mice were compared, serum IgG obtained from animals vaccinated with TIV complexed with sFc IgG showed significantly increased binding to the H1 from several other strains, and H3 and even H5 from avian influenza virus. This showed that IC elicited higher-affinity antibody responses that were enhanced for breadth and potency of activity against influenza viruses in mice. In some settings, a Fc point mutation F241A could function in place of the sialylation to engage CD23, ICs produced with this antibody also demonstrated high potency in inducing neutralizing antibodies again HA (Maamary et al. 2017). This observation has significant implication in practical deployment for development of an universal seasonal flu vaccine. Also in TIV vaccination, ICs may play a role in NK cell-mediated ADCC. In TIV recipients, plasma sera collected from those patients facilitated NK cell degranulation in the presence of TIV, suggesting an IC-dependent cytolytic event (Goodier et al. 2016).

Another modified version of IC was to fuse the Fc fragment with a specific antigen. This has been explored in H5N1 vaccine, an influenza A subtype virus that surfaced in 2003 and has been circulating in aves and spreading to humans with severe morbidity and high mortality. Although a number of preventive vaccines against H5N1 have been studied in mice (Biesova et al. 2009; Szecsi et al. 2009; Tao et al. 2009), and in preclinical evaluation (Kreijtz et al. 2009), Du et al. developed a new approach and designed two recombinant influenza vaccine candidates by fusing HA1 fragment of A/Anhui/1/2005(H5N1) to either Fc of human IgG (HA1-Fc) or foldon plus Fc (HA1-Fdc). Both proteins were able to induce high titer of antibodies. Importantly, immunization with these two vaccine candidates, especially HA1-Fdc, provided complete cross-clade protection against high-dose lethal challenge of different strains of H5N1 virus covering clade 0, 1 and 2.3.4 in mouse model. This finding suggests that fusing HA antigen with Fc could be developed into an efficacious universal H5N1 influenza vaccine (Du et al. 2011).

ICs have been used to enhance flu-specific cytolytic T cells in special populations. CTL response in aging populations has reduced potency. In young Balb/c mice, although NP-specific CTL response can be readily induced with either killed H1N1 virus or in combination with a NP-specific antibody, only the latter was able trigger strong cytolytic response in older mice. This enhanced killing was accompanied by strong IFN-γ secretion by both CD8 and CD4 T cells (Zheng et al. 2007). Although these experiments point to specific use of ICs in influenza virus protection, the advantages demonstrated may be important in setting up larger scale prophylactic vaccination for other viral infections.

3.3   IC Vaccination for HIV Infection

HIV, an RNA retrovirus, enters cellular nucleus for genome integration during host cell replication cycle. Although HIV was discovered several decades ago, due to its long latent period, several transmission modes and lifelong persistency, AIDS is still at the top of global medical concerns. Currently, antiretroviral drugs have been effective in prolonging the life span of AIDS patients and reducing the mortality, yet morbidity of AIDS in some developing countries and burden of health care cost are still great concerns. From epidemiological prospective, effective prophylactic HIV vaccine remains the most desirable measure. Currently, DNA-based vaccines with prime and boost strategy, new/altered delivery protocols as well as approaches to rebuild the damaged host immune systems are under study (Chen et al. 2014).

Initial attempts of IC-based HIV vaccination were not all successful. Adenovirus 5 (Ad5) encoding HIV epitopes in complex with anti adeno antibodies have been tested in clinical trials (Shiver and Emini 2004). In a preliminary study, adeno vector carrying β galactosidase sequence was used in combination of antibody targeting the vector. Although the higher antibody to virus ratio induced a transient T cell response and little humoral response, a lower ratio was effective in triggering both arms of immunity against the model antigen (Choi et al. 2012). Importantly, the presence of antibody significantly reduced the toxic effect of the viral vector. In the STEP trials, HIV *gag*, *pol* and *nef* gene cassettes were inserted into the adeno vector, however individuals with preexisting immunity against the vector showed greater risk of HIV infection following the immunization (Buchbinder et al. 2008). Subsequent studies indicated that likely due to mucosal localization of Ad5 viral accumulation, a T cell response characterized by high α4β7 and CCR9 expression was detected, coupled with higher CCR5 (HIV co-receptor) level. In addition, adeno virus-stimulated T cells were more susceptible to HIV entry, aggravating the risk of vaccine recipients (Benlahrech et al. 2009; Perreau et al. 2008). In a rhesus monkey model, a non-neutralizing antibody against SIV did not significantly protect the recipients from secondary challenges in comparison with the SIV immunization alone (Polyanskaya et al. 2001). In fact, anti-gp41 antibody resulted in IC that was associated with FcγRIIB signaling, and in expression of anti-inflammatory genes such as SPRED1 and COMMD1, likely to suppress immune responses.

In other attempts, IC-based vaccines for HIV were reported by scientists using antibodies recognizing CD4-binding sites and V3 region of gp120, which has shown to elicit neutralizing antibodies in mice (Hioe et al. 2009; Visciano et al. 2008). As the variances in gp120 are large, a monoclonal antibody (654-D) with high affinity to a large number of V3 variants was found, and the ICs formed using this antibody induced V3 neutralizing antibodies in Balb/c mice (Hioe et al. 2009). Interestingly, binding by this antibody exposed other epitopes in the V3 that are usually inaccessible by other mAb. Similarly, IC formed with mAb A32 that binds to gp120 also induced neutralizing antibodies against a number of HIV strains (Liao et al. 2004). This strategy of "induced accessibility" offers a new concept in the clinical use of ICs as anti-viral treatments.

The concept of broadly neutralizing antibodies (bNAbs) against HIV is the most intensely studied AIDS treatment at the moment. High-throughput screening of B cells from HIV carriers has identified clones that are capable of targeting multiple HIV subtypes (Walker et al. 2009; Wu et al. 2010). For AIDS treatment, the strategy employed to reactivate the latent virus with antiretroviral treatment followed by immune therapies is also under trial. bNAbs are usually effective in controlling HIV viremia in mice (Horwitz et al. 2013). However, one important concern is the viremia rebound following the termination of treatment. One way to combat this problem is to use multiple bNAbs at the same time, i.e., TriMix antibodies (3BNC117, anti-CD4bs; PG16, anti-V1/V2 loop region; and 10-1074, anti-V3) that can significantly delay the rebound. The other strategy is the "shock and kill" that involves the use of TriMix in combination with several viral inducers. This can suppress the rebound for several months (Halper-Stromberg et al. 2014). It is important to note that the control TriMix carrying mutated Fc that is unable to engage FcγRs has a reduced inhibition of the viremia reappearance. Fc swapping analysis suggested that for a given Fab, mouse IgG2A Fc has the highest potency in blocking HIV. In a mouse model whereby human FcγRs were used to genetically replace mouse counterparts, human IgG1 carrying mutations that facilitate binding to activating FcγRs (FcγRIIA and FcγRIIIA) was more effective comparing with the mutations that abolish the binding (Bournazos et al. 2014).

In SIV and SHIV (Simian HIV is a chimeric virus in which HIV Env substitutes for that of SIV) models, ICs formed with infected cells were more efficiently captured by DCs than infected cells alone, leading to stronger functional DC activation, potent anti-viral cytotoxic T lymphocyte and T cell memory responses and the inhibition of the expansion of regulatory T cells (Lambour et al. 2016; Pelegrin et al. 2015). One mouse model has drawn great interest in studying human vertical HIV transmission in childbearing mothers. FcCasE virus-infected mice during pregnancy can transmit the virus to the newborn. This infection causes erythroleukemia once the offspring reach the adulthood. Neonatal injection of mAb 66 induced both antibody and T cell responses against the virus and significantly increased the rate of long survival in comparison with the nearly total fatality in the untreated (Michaud et al. 2010).

3.4 IC Vaccination for Viral Hepatitis B

Hepatitis B virus (HBV) belongs to hepadnaviridae, a DNA virus which replicates via a RNA–DNA intermediate. HBV enters cell nucleus forming an episomal closed covalent circular DNA (cccDNA). cccDNA is replenished by recycling of the viral genome and is the template for transcription and translation of multiple viral proteins: Hepatitis B surface antigen (HBsAg), Hepatitis core antigen (HBcAg) and the viral polymerase. Translational modification of HBcAg generates a secreted protein HBeAg, which is a marker for the replication of virus (Seeger and Mason 2015). Despite the remarkable success of prophylactic hepatitis B vaccines, there are still around 300 million HBsAg-positive carriers worldwide. Among them, some will progress to chronic hepatitis B (CHB), liver cirrhosis and hepatocellular carcinoma. Multiple immune defects have been revealed in chronic CHB patients (Schmidt et al. 2013) and restoration of effective host immune responses is necessary for virus clearance.

Currently, several therapeutic vaccines for CHB are in experimental or clinical studies (Lobaina and Michel 2017). Based on our previous approach of using ICs absorbed to SMAA for restoration of immune responses in duck hepatitis B virus-infected immune tolerant ducks (Wen et al. 1994), a YIC (yeast-derived recombinant HBsAg complexed to human anti-HBsAg antibody) therapeutic vaccine candidate for CHB patients has been developed. We hypothesized that due to the persistence of huge amount of HBV antigens, CHB patients are immune tolerant and cannot generate effective immune responses against the virus, as a part of immune defects in the carriers. HBsAg complexed with its antibodies was expected to activate APCs to uptake ICs through their FcγRs, and the antigen will be processed and presented effectively to T cells (Wen 2009). In vitro studies with PBMCs stimulated with GM-CSF/IL-4 from CHB patients, HBsAg-anti-HBs upregulated HLA-II, CD80, CD86 and CD40 molecules on DCs and improved dendritic and T cell interactions as measured by IFN-γ and IL-2 production (Yao et al. 2007). One version of HBsAg ICs was able to induce antibody production in HBsAg-transgenic mice, followed by a seroconversion to become HBsAg positive (Celis et al. 1987; Zheng et al. 2001). HBsAg Fc fusion protein was also able to enhance T cell cytotoxicity and to decrease serum HBsAg in HBsAg-transgenic mice (Meng et al. 2012). These efforts were followed up by clinical trials.

Although a number of HBV vaccines are in clinical trials (Lobaina and Michel 2017), the IC-based therapeutic vaccine is leading in many aspects. In a pilot study, HBsAg IC mixed with alum was used in HBV carriers and reached statistically significant reduction in blood HBV DNA (Wen et al. 1995). YIC was approved by China FDA for clinical trial in 2002 and is currently entering phase III. In phase I trial among healthy adults, YIC induced high titer of anti-HBs and up-regulated production of IL-2 and IFN-γ (Xu et al. 2005). Subsequently, in phase II A and B clinical trials, a decrease in serum viral load and seroconversion from serum HBeAg positive to anti-HBe positive were observed, with cytolytic and noncytolytic immune responses comparable to treatment with conventional IFNα. To analyze the cellular immune responses induced by YIC, a pilot study in patients treated with this IC and the controls (alum and saline) were studied together with an anti-HBV drug, adefovir, as a basic treatment. Results showed that the relative number of specific CD4 and CD8 T cells were increased with decrease of Treg cells in patients treated with YIC, compared to those in the control groups (Zhou et al. 2017). These clinical observations correlated well with results previously observed in vitro and in mice, indicating that ICs are a promising therapeutic vaccine for treatment of CHB patients.

Recently, several human anti-HB neutralizing antibodies for treatment of animal models mimicking CHB were reported. One antibody (2H5-A14) that blocks viral large envelop protein preS1 domain binding to its receptor sodium taurocholate cotransporting polypeptide was highly neutralizing. 2H5-A14 therapeutic effect was dependent on FcγRs (Li et al. 2017). In another model, mAb E6F6 binding to a conserved epitope on the virion resulted in formation of ICs and FcγR-dependent phagocytosis. E6F6 treatment blocked HBV infection and restored anti-HBV T cell responses in carrier mice (Zhang et al. 2016). In an HBV hydrodynamic injected mouse model, another broadly neutralizing human monoclonal antibody against HBsAg, G12, was shown to decrease mouse serum HbsAg, with a potency 1000 times higher than that of the current HBIG (Wang et al. 2016). These new findings offer more diverse approaches of applying ICs in HBV prevention and treatment.

3.5 IC Vaccination for Tumors

Antibodies have long been considered a valid approach in cancer treatment. The most discussed and so far the most successful intervention is to use antibodies or their derivatives to block negative signaling such as CTLA4 and PD1/PDL1 in immune cells, better known as check point blockage. Another category of antibody-based cancer therapy involves inhibition of growth factors such as VEGF and EGFR (Nimmerjahn and Ravetch 2012). IC-based therapies in comparison are at the experimental stage. However, the inherent safety and better patient toleration make this class of treatments a worthwhile study topic.

Antibody-based immune therapies can be divided into direct cell death induction and immune responses against tumor as consequence of immunization. Some antibodies against tumor surface molecules can induce FcγR-dependent ADCC, leading to tumor cell apoptosis (Moalli et al. 2010). ICs in this setting have shown greater flexibility and can be used for prophylactic and therapeutic intervention. A well-studied mouse model is B16 melanoma expressing transfected OVA antigen. For instance, in an OVA-expressing B16 tumor inoculation model, injection of DCs pulsed with OVA ICs inhibited the tumor. In fact, it reached a 40% eradication of the established tumor in mice. The ICs induced memory responses in mice that were protective in secondary tumor challenges (Rafiq et al. 2002).

The IC-based anti-tumor treatment has been tested with real-life tumor antigens. Antibodies against tumor antigens such as HER2/neu and syndecan-1 triggered strong CD8 T cell responses against the antigen-bearing tumors. These effects were mainly mediated via facilitated antigen presentation (Dhodapkar et al. 2002; Kim et al. 2008; Wolpoe et al. 2003). Tumor antigen Syndecan-1-specific antibody-treated melanoma stimulated HLA-A2.1-restricted cytolytic T cell response against some of the best-known tumor antigens such as MAGE-3 and NY-Eso-1, suggesting targeting one antigen can release sufficient bystander activation of T cells against epitopes otherwise "unseen" by the immune system (Dhodapkar et al. 2002).

While there is no doubt that in the IC-based tumor therapy models FcγRs were involved both at opsonization/phagocytosis and DC maturation, an emerging consideration is the ratio of engagement of activating and inhibitory FcγRs (Nimmerjahn and Ravetch 2005). Although historically the involvement of antibody subtypes and FcγRs was not a carefully controlled aspect, Ravetch et al. suggested that proper matching of Fcs with their activating and inhibitory receptors could be used to induce preferred anti-tumor effects (Nimmerjahn and Ravetch 2005). mIgG2A subtype antibody TA99 binds to activating FcγRs with high affinity. If the binding was targeted to FcγRIV, a strong anti-tumor effect was observed (Nimmerjahn and Ravetch 2005). Their group also reported that CD20-specific IgG2A antibody treatment led to prolonged survival of mice challenged with CD20-positive EL4 cells. In this setup, mice with a DC-specific deletion of FcγRIV were not protected by the same treatment (DiLillo and Ravetch 2015). Future efforts in precise engineering to select proper activating/inhibitory ratio in IgG subtype/FcγR pairs likely represent some of the best options in IC-based cancer treatment.

The role of ICs in tumor therapies may be unintentionally built into some existing protocols. Several reports have shown that the antibodies against TNF family receptors, such as OX40 as well as CTLA4, intensely studied in check point therapy, in fact depleted Tregs in vivo in an activating FcγR-dependent manner (Bulliard et al. 2013; Bulliard et al. 2014; Simpson et al. 2013). In another instance, Imprime, a glucan like anti-tumor drug intended to induce innate immune responses, required serum anti β-glucan antibodies (ABA) to achieve its effects in patients. ABA binding to Imprime resulted in complement fixation, ROS production and antibody-dependent phagocytosis. In patients with low existing ABA, provision of ABA increased the innate immune responses (Chan et al. 2016). Such "unintended" effects mediated by ICs are worthwhile topics for a variety of current cancer treatment protocols.

4   Future Prospective of IC Vaccines

In the development of IC vaccines, the goal remains to be the induction of a broad spectrum of neutralizing antibodies against a microbe or a tumor antigen along with a well-developed cell-mediated immunity. Such efforts are currently seeing a great deal of success in IC-based treatments of HIV and influenza virus infections. For future development, it is important to obtain similar efficacies to other viruses, particularly those causing prevalent infections in humans and livestock. Although approaches can be multifaceted, it appears that the leading research should be centered on bNAbs and proper matching of Fc subtypes to induce activation of a desired ratio of inhibitory and activating FcγRs.

Several fronts in technology development are opening up new territories for IC vaccines. Yoshida et al. reported that FcRn is the vehicle that transports IgG across the intestinal epithelial barrier into the lumen. This transportation delivers IgG/ antigen complex into the lamina propria for processing by DCs and presentation to CD4+ T cells in regional lymphoid structures (Yoshida et al. 2004). This suggests that IC vaccines could be delivered via the oral route. This possibility was confirmed by a pilot experiment of HBsAg IC immunization *per os* in mice (our unpublished results). Another important function of FcRn is the transcytosis of IgG in the placental syncytiotrophoblasts. As maternal vaccination becomes an increasingly important strategy for the protection of young infants, employing ICs via FcRn for pregnant women may be considered in low-income countries where the burden of infant morbidity and mortality is highest (Chu and Englund 2014; Yoshida et al. 2004). Another area that deserves particular attention is the new technologies applied in understanding, identifying and designing most efficacious antigen specificity determinants (Fabs) with broad coverage on intended pathogens. Efforts are being made to introduce a set of "common principles" based on molecular, genetic and structural knowledge to generate most cutting-edge antibody treatment (Crowe 2017). These principles are almost certainly applicable in IC-based therapies.

Although IC vaccination has a long history, its application in preventive and therapeutic clinical trials is still at an early stage. Sustained exploration of mechanisms of IC vaccines by basic research scientists, objective and candid evaluations on clinical trials by clinicians, ample financial support from industries, and comprehensive and systematic guidelines from regulatory authorities are all indispensable in a joint effort to bring this technology to its fruition for public health benefits.

Acknowledgements YM. W. has been supported by 863 Grants from China National Science and Technology since 1988–2008, and supported by the Grand Research Program for Infectious Diseases, China (2008ZX10002-003, 2012ZX10002002004, 2017ZX10202201002.

Y. S. is supported by the joint Peking-Tsinghua Center for Life Sciences, the National Natural Science Foundation of China General Program (31370878), and by grants from the US NIH (R01AI098995), the Natural Sciences and Engineering Research Council of Canada (RGPIN-355350/396037) and the Canadian Institutes for Health Research (MOP-119295).

References

Amigorena S, Bonnerot C (1999) Fc receptors for IgG and antigen presentation on MHC class I and class II molecules. Semin Immunol 11:385–390

Benlahrech A, Harris J, Meiser A, Papagatsias T, Hornig J, Hayes P, Lieber A, Athanasopoulos T, Bachy V, Csomor E, Daniels R, Fisher K, Gotch F, Seymour L, Logan K, Barbagallo R, Klavinskis L, Dickson G, Patterson S (2009) Adenovirus vector vaccination induces expansion of memory CD4 T cells with a mucosal homing phenotype that are readily susceptible to HIV-1. Proc Natl Acad Sci U S A 106:19940–19945

Bergtold A, Desai DD, Gavhane A, Clynes R (2005) Cell surface recycling of internalized antigen permits dendritic cell priming of B cells. Immunity 23:503–514

Berken A, Benacerraf B (1966) Properties of antibodies cytophilic for macrophages. J Exp Med 123:119–144

Berlyn KA, Schultes B, Leveugle B, Noujaim AA, Alexander RB, Mann DL (2001) Generation of CD4(+) and CD8(+) T lymphocyte responses by dendritic cells armed with PSA/anti-PSA (antigen/antibody) complexes. Clin Immunol 101:276–283

Berzofsky JA, Bensussan A, Cease KB, Bourge JF, Cheynier R, Lurhuma Z, Salaun JJ, Gallo RC, Shearer GM, Zagury D (1988) Antigenic peptides recognized by T lymphocytes from AIDS viral envelope-immune humans. Nature 334:706–708

Bevan MJ (1976) Cross-priming for a secondary cytotoxic response to minor H antigens with H-2 congenic cells which do not cross-react in the cytotoxic assay. J Exp Med 143:1283–1288

Biesova Z, Miller MA, Schneerson R, Shiloach J, Green KY, Robbins JB, Keith JM (2009) Preparation, characterization, and immunogenicity in mice of a recombinant influenza H5 hemagglutinin vaccine against the avian H5N1 A/Vietnam/1203/2004 influenza virus. Vaccine 27:6234–6238

Boesch AW, Brown EP, Cheng HD, Ofori MO, Normandin E, Nigrovic PA, Alter G, Ackerman ME (2014) Highly parallel characterization of IgG Fc binding interactions. MAbs 6:915–927

Boross P, van Montfoort N, Stapels DA, van der Poel CE, Bertens C, Meeldijk J, Jansen JH, Verbeek JS, Ossendorp F, Wubbolts R, Leusen JH (2014) FcRgamma-chain ITAM signaling is critically required for cross-presentation of soluble antibody-antigen complexes by dendritic cells. J Immunol 193:5506–5514

Bournazos S, DiLillo DJ, Ravetch JV (2015) The role of Fc-FcgammaR interactions in IgG-mediated microbial neutralization. J Exp Med 212:1361–1369

Bournazos S, Klein F, Pietzsch J, Seaman MS, Nussenzweig MC, Ravetch JV (2014) Broadly neutralizing anti-HIV-1 antibodies require Fc effector functions for in vivo activity. Cell 158:1243–1253

Boyden SV, Sorkin E (1960) The adsorption of antigen by spleen cells previously treated with antiserum in vitro. Immunology 3:272–283

Bruhns P (2012) Properties of mouse and human IgG receptors and their contribution to disease models. Blood 119:5640–5649

Buchbinder SP, Mehrotra DV, Duerr A, Fitzgerald DW, Mogg R, Li D, Gilbert PB, Lama JR, Marmor M, Del Rio C, McElrath MJ, Casimiro DR, Gottesdiener KM, Chodakewitz JA, Corey L, Robertson MN, Step Study Protocol Team (2008) Efficacy assessment of a cell-mediated immunity HIV-1 vaccine (the Step Study): a double-blind, randomised, placebo-controlled, test-of-concept trial. Lancet 372:1881–1893

Bulliard Y, Jolicoeur R, Windman M, Rue SM, Ettenberg S, Knee DA, Wilson NS, Dranoff G, Brogdon JL (2013) Activating Fc gamma receptors contribute to the antitumor activities of immunoregulatory receptor-targeting antibodies. J Exp Med 210:1685–1693

Bulliard Y, Jolicoeur R, Zhang J, Dranoff G, Wilson N, Brogdon J (2014) OX40 engagement depletes intratumoral Tregs via activating FcγRs, leading to antitumor efficacy. Immunol Cell Biol 92

Burgdorf S, Kautz A, Bohnert V, Knolle PA, Kurts C (2007) Distinct pathways of antigen uptake and intracellular routing in CD4 and CD8 T cell activation. Science 316:612–616

Celis E, Abraham KG, Miller RW (1987) Modulation of the immunological response to hepatitis B virus by antibodies. Hepatology 7:563–568

Celis E, Chang TW (1984) Antibodies to hepatitis B surface antigen potentiate the response of human T lymphocyte clones to the same antigen. Science 224:297–299

Celis E, Zurawski VR Jr, Chang TW (1984) Regulation of T-cell function by antibodies: enhancement of the response of human T-cell clones to hepatitis B surface antigen by antigen-specific monoclonal antibodies. Proc Natl Acad Sci U S A 81:6846–6850

Cendrowski J, Maminska A, Miaczynska M (2016) Endocytic regulation of cytokine receptor signaling. Cytokine Growth Factor Rev 32:63–73

Chan AS, Jonas AB, Qiu X, Ottoson NR, Walsh RM, Gorden KB, Harrison B, Maimonis PJ, Leonardo SM, Ertelt KE, Danielson ME, Michel KS, Nelson M, Graff JR, Patchen ML, Bose N (2016) Imprime PGG-mediated anti-cancer immune activation requires immune complex formation. PLoS One 11:e0165909

Chatterjee B, Smed-Sorensen A, Cohn L, Chalouni C, Vandlen R, Lee BC, Widger J, Keler T, Delamarre L, Mellman I (2012) Internalization and endosomal degradation of receptor-bound antigens regulate the efficiency of cross presentation by human dendritic cells. Blood 120:2011–2020

Chen Y, Wang S, Lu S (2014) DNA immunization for HIV vaccine development. Vaccines 2:138–159

Choi JH, Dekker J, Schafer SC, John J, Whitfill CE, Petty CS, Haddad EE, Croyle MA (2012) Optimized adenovirus-antibody complexes stimulate strong cellular and humoral immune responses against an encoded antigen in naive mice and those with preexisting immunity. Clin Vaccine Immunol 19:84–95

Chu HY, Englund JA (2014) Maternal immunization. Clin Infect Dis 59:560–568

Clatworthy MR, Aronin CE, Mathews RJ, Morgan NY, Smith KG, Germain RN (2014) Immune complexes stimulate CCR7-dependent dendritic cell migration to lymph nodes. Nat Med 20:1458–1463

Cohn L, Chatterjee B, Esselborn F, Smed-Sorensen A, Nakamura N, Chalouni C, Lee BC, Vandlen R, Keler T, Lauer P, Brockstedt D, Mellman I, Delamarre L (2013) Antigen delivery to early endosomes eliminates the superiority of human blood BDCA3+ dendritic cells at cross presentation. J Exp Med 210:1049–1063

Copeman SM, O'brien RA, Eagleton AJ, Glenny AT (1922) Experiences with the schick test and active immunization against diphtheria. Brit J Exper Path 3:42

Crowe JE Jr (2017) Principles of broad and potent antiviral human antibodies: insights for vaccine design. Cell Host Microbe 22:193–206

de Jong JM, Schuurhuis DH, Ioan-Facsinay A, Welling MM, Camps MG, van der Voort EI, Huizinga TW, Ossendorp F, Verbeek JS, Toes RE (2006) Dendritic cells, but not macrophages or B cells, activate major histocompatibility complex class II-restricted CD4+ T cells upon immune-complex uptake in vivo. Immunology 119:499–506

den Haan JM, Bevan MJ (2002) Constitutive versus activation-dependent cross-presentation of immune complexes by CD8(+) and CD8(−) dendritic cells in vivo. J Exp Med 196:817–827

Dhodapkar KM, Krasovsky J, Williamson B, Dhodapkar MV (2002) Antitumor monoclonal antibodies enhance cross-presentation of cellular antigens and the generation of myeloma-specific killer T cells by dendritic cells. J Exp Med 195:125–133

DiLillo DJ, Ravetch JV (2015) Differential Fc-receptor engagement drives an anti-tumor vaccinal effect. Cell 161:1035–1045

Du L, Leung VH-C, Zhang X, Zhou J, Chen M, He W, Zhang H-Y, Chan CCS, Poon VK-M, Zhao G, Sun S, Cai L, Zhou Y, Zheng B-J, Jiang S (2011) A recombinant vaccine of H5N1 HA1 fused with foldon and human IgG Fc induced complete cross-clade protection against divergent H5N1 viruses. PLoS ONE 6:e16555

Goodier MR, Lusa C, Sherratt S, Rodriguez-Galan A, Behrens R, Riley EM (2016) Sustained immune complex-mediated reduction in CD16 expression after vaccination regulates NK cell function. Front Immunol 7:384

Gosselin EJ, Bitsaktsis C, Li Y, Iglesias BV (2009) Fc receptor-targeted mucosal vaccination as a novel strategy for the generation of enhanced immunity against mucosal and non-mucosal pathogens. Arch Immunol Ther Exp (Warsz) 57:311–323

Haddad EE, Whitfill CE, Avakian AP, Ricks CA, Andrews PD, Thoma JA, Wakenell PS (1997) Efficacy of a novel infectious bursal disease virus immune complex vaccine in broiler chickens. Avian Diseases 41:882–889

Halper-Stromberg A, Lu CL, Klein F, Horwitz JA, Bournazos S, Nogueira L, Eisenreich TR, Liu C, Gazumyan A, Schaefer U, Furze RC, Seaman MS, Prinjha R, Tarakhovsky A, Ravetch JV, Nussenzweig MC (2014) Broadly neutralizing antibodies and viral inducers decrease rebound from HIV-1 latent reservoirs in humanized mice. Cell 158:989–999

Harbers SO, Crocker A, Catalano G, D'Agati V, Jung S, Desai DD, Clynes R (2007) Antibody-enhanced cross-presentation of self antigen breaks T cell tolerance. J Clin Invest 117:1361–1369

Hari A, Ganguly A, Mu L, Davis SP, Stenner MD, Lam R, Munro F, Namet I, Alghamdi E, Furstenhaupt T, Dong W, Detampel P, Shen LJ, Amrein MW, Yates RM, Shi Y (2015) Redirecting soluble antigen for MHC class I cross-presentation during phagocytosis. Eur J Immunol 45:383–395

Heesters BA, Chatterjee P, Kim YA, Gonzalez SF, Kuligowski MP, Kirchhausen T, Carroll MC (2013) Endocytosis and recycling of immune complexes by follicular dendritic cells enhances B cell antigen binding and activation. Immunity 38:1164–1175

Hioe CE, Visciano ML, Kumar R, Liu J, Mack EA, Simon RE, Levy DN, Tuen M (2009) The use of immune complex vaccines to enhance antibody responses against neutralizing epitopes on HIV-1 envelope gp120. Vaccine 28:352–360

Horwitz JA, Halper-Stromberg A, Mouquet H, Gitlin AD, Tretiakova A, Eisenreich TR, Malbec M, Gravemann S, Billerbeck E, Dorner M, Buning H, Schwartz O, Knops E, Kaiser R, Seaman MS, Wilson JM, Rice CM, Ploss A, Bjorkman PJ, Klein F, Nussenzweig MC (2013) HIV-1 suppression and durable control by combining single broadly neutralizing antibodies and antiretroviral drugs in humanized mice. Proc Natl Acad Sci U S A 110:16538–16543

Ignjatovic J, Gould G, Trinidad L, Sapats S (2006) Chicken recombinant antibodies against infectious bursal disease virus are able to form antibody-virus immune complex. Avian Pathol 35:293–301

Iván J, Velhner M, Ursu K, Germán P, Mató T, Drén CN, Mészáros J (2005) Delayed vaccine virus replication in chickens vaccinated subcutaneously with an immune complex infectious bursal disease vaccine: Quantification of vaccine virus by real-time polymerase chain reaction. Can J Vet Res 69:135–142

Jeurissen SH, Janse EM, Lehrbach PR, Haddad EE, Avakian A, Whitfill CE (1998) The working mechanism of an immune complex vaccine that protects chickens against infectious bursal disease. Immunology 95:494–500

Joffre OP, Segura E, Savina A, Amigorena S (2012) Cross-presentation by dendritic cells. Nat Rev Immunol 12:557–569

Kapczynski DR, Afonso CL, Miller PJ (2013) Immune responses of poultry to Newcastle disease virus. Dev Comp Immunol 41:447–453

Kim PS, Armstrong TD, Song H, Wolpoe ME, Weiss V, Manning EA, Huang LQ, Murata S, Sgouros G, Emens LA, Reilly RT, Jaffee EM (2008) Antibody association with HER-2/neu-targeted vaccine enhances CD8 T cell responses in mice through Fc-mediated activation of DCs. J Clin Invest 118:1700–1711

Kool M, Fierens K, Lambrecht BN (2012) Alum adjuvant: some of the tricks of the oldest adjuvant. J Med Microbiol 61:927–934

Kosco MH, Burton GF, Kapasi ZF, Szakal AK, Tew JG (1989) Antibody-forming cell induction during an early phase of germinal centre development and its delay with ageing. Immunology 68:312–318

Kreijtz JH, Suezer Y, de Mutsert G, van den Brand JM, van Amerongen G, Schnierle BS, Kuiken T, Fouchier RA, Lower J, Osterhaus AD, Sutter G, Rimmelzwaan GF (2009) Preclinical evaluation of a modified vaccinia virus Ankara (MVA)-based vaccine against influenza A/H5N1 viruses. Vaccine 27:6296–6299

Lambour J, Naranjo-Gomez M, Piechaczyk M, Pelegrin M (2016) Converting monoclonal antibody-based immunotherapies from passive to active: bringing immune complexes into play. Emer Microbes & Infect 5:e92

Le Roux D, Lankar D, Yuseff MI, Vascotto F, Yokozeki T, Faure-Andre G, Mougneau E, Glaichenhaus N, Manoury B, Bonnerot C, Lennon-Dumenil AM (2007) Syk-dependent actin dynamics regulate endocytic trafficking and processing of antigens internalized through the B-cell receptor. Mol Biol Cell 18:3451–3462

Lehmann CHK, Baranska A, Heidkamp GF, Heger L, Neubert K, Lühr JJ, Hoffmann A, Reimer KC, Brückner C, Beck S, Seeling M, Kießling M, Soulat D, Krug AB, Ravetch JV,

Leusen JHW, Nimmerjahn F, Dudziak D (2017) DC subset–specific induction of T cell responses upon antigen uptake via Fcγ receptors in vivo. J Exper Med 214:1509–1528

Leon B, Ballesteros-Tato A, Randall TD, Lund FE (2014) Prolonged antigen presentation by immune complex-binding dendritic cells programs the proliferative capacity of memory CD8 T cells. J Exp Med 211:1637–1655

Li D, He W, Liu X, Zheng S, Qi Y, Li H, Mao F, Liu J, Sun Y, Pan L, Du K, Ye K, Li W, Sui J (2017) A potent human neutralizing antibody Fc-dependently reduces established HBV infections. eLife 6:e26738

Li Q, Zeng M, Duan L, Voss JE, Smith AJ, Pambuccian S, Shang L, Wietgrefe S, Southern PJ, Reilly CS, Skinner PJ, Zupancic ML, Carlis JV, Piatak M Jr, Waterman D, Reeves RK, Masek-Hammerman K, Derdeyn CA, Alpert MD, Evans DT, Kohler H, Muller S, Robinson J, Lifson JD, Burton DR, Johnson RP, Haase AT (2014) Live simian immunodeficiency virus vaccine correlate of protection: local antibody production and concentration on the path of virus entry. J Immunol 193:3113–3125

Liao HX, Alam SM, Mascola JR, Robinson J, Ma B, Montefiori DC, Rhein M, Sutherland LL, Scearce R, Haynes BF (2004) Immunogenicity of constrained monoclonal antibody A32-human immunodeficiency virus (HIV) Env gp120 complexes compared to that of recombinant HIV type 1 gp120 envelope glycoproteins. J Virol 78:5270–5278

Lizee G, Basha G, Tiong J, Julien JP, Tian M, Biron KE, Jefferies WA (2003) Control of dendritic cell cross-presentation by the major histocompatibility complex class I cytoplasmic domain. Nat Immunol 4:1065–1073

Lobaina Y, Michel ML (2017) Chronic hepatitis B: Immunological profile and current therapeutic vaccines in clinical trials. Vaccine 35:2308–2314

Lux A, Yu X, Scanlan CN, Nimmerjahn F (2013) Impact of immune complex size and glycosylation on IgG binding to human FcgammaRs. J Immunol 190:4315–4323

Maamary J, Wang TT, Tan GS, Palese P, Ravetch JV (2017) Increasing the breadth and potency of response to the seasonal influenza virus vaccine by immune complex immunization. Proc Natl Acad Sci U S A 114:10172–10177

Marois L, Pare G, Vaillancourt M, Rollet-Labelle E, Naccache PH (2011) Fc gammaRIIIb triggers raft-dependent calcium influx in IgG-mediated responses in human neutrophils. J Biol Chem 286:3509–3519

Matsubara S, Koya T, Takeda K, Joetham A, Miyahara N, Pine P, Masuda ES, Swasey CH, Gelfand EW (2006) Syk activation in dendritic cells is essential for airway hyperresponsiveness and inflammation. Am J Respir Cell Mol Biol 34:426–433

McEwan WA, Tam JC, Watkinson RE, Bidgood SR, Mallery DL, James LC (2013) Intracellular antibody-bound pathogens stimulate immune signaling via the Fc receptor TRIM21. Nat Immunol 14:327–336

Meng ZF, Wang HJ, Yao X, Wang XY, Wen YM, Dai JX, Xie YH, Xu JQ (2012) Immunization with HBsAg-Fc fusion protein induces a predominant production of Th1 cytokines and reduces HBsAg level in transgenic mice. Chin Med J (Engl) 125:3266–3272

Mi W, Wanjie S, Lo ST, Gan Z, Pickl-Herk B, Ober RJ, Ward ES (2008) Targeting the neonatal fc receptor for antigen delivery using engineered fc fragments. J Immunol 181:7550–7561

Michaud HA, Gomard T, Gros L, Thiolon K, Nasser R, Jacquet C, Hernandez J, Piechaczyk M, Pelegrin M (2010) A crucial role for infected-cell/antibody immune complexes in the enhancement of endogenous antiviral immunity by short passive immunotherapy. PLoS Pathog 6:e1000948

Moalli F, Doni A, Deban L, Zelante T, Zagarella S, Bottazzi B, Romani L, Mantovani A, Garlanda C (2010) Role of complement and Fc{gamma} receptors in the protective activity of the long pentraxin PTX3 against Aspergillus fumigatus. Blood 116:5170–5180

Mocsai A, Ruland J, Tybulewicz VL (2010) The SYK tyrosine kinase: a crucial player in diverse biological functions. Nat Rev Immunol 10:387–402

Morrison SL, Terres G (1966) Enhanced immunologic sensitization of mice by the simultaneous injection of antigen and specific antiserum. II. Effect of varying the antigen-antibody ratio and the amount of immune complex injected. J Immunol 96:901–905

Müller H, Mundt E, Eterradossi N, Islam MR (2012) Current status of vaccines against infectious bursal disease. Avian Pathology 41:133–139

Naqi SA, Marquez B, Sahin N (1983) Maternal antibody and its effect on infectious bursal disease immunization. Avian Dis 27:623–631

Nimmerjahn F, Bruhns P, Horiuchi K, Ravetch JV (2005) FcgammaRIV: a novel FcR with distinct IgG subclass specificity. Immunity 23:41–51

Nimmerjahn F, Ravetch JV (2005) Divergent immunoglobulin g subclass activity through selective Fc receptor binding. Science 310:1510–1512

Nimmerjahn F, Ravetch JV (2012) Translating basic mechanisms of IgG effector activity into next generation cancer therapies. Cancer Immun 12:13

Oefner CM, Winkler A, Hess C, Lorenz AK, Holecska V, Huxdorf M, Schommartz T, Petzold D, Bitterling J, Schoen AL, Stoehr AD, Van Vu D, Darcan-Nikolaisen Y, Blanchard V, Schmudde I, Laumonnier Y, Strover HA, Hegazy AN, Eiglmeier S, Schoen CT, Mertes MM, Loddenkemper C, Lohning M, Konig P, Petersen A, Luger EO, Collin M, Kohl J, Hutloff A, Hamelmann E, Berger M, Wardemann H, Ehlers M (2012) Tolerance induction with T cell-dependent protein antigens induces regulatory sialylated IgGs. J Allergy Clin Immunol 129(1647–1655):e1613

Park-Min KH, Serbina NV, Yang W, Ma X, Krystal G, Neel BG, Nutt SL, Hu X, Ivashkiv LB (2007) FcgammaRIII-dependent inhibition of interferon-gamma responses mediates suppressive effects of intravenous immune globulin. Immunity 26:67–78

Pelegrin M, Naranjo-Gomez M, Piechaczyk M (2015) Antiviral monoclonal antibodies: can they be more than simple neutralizing agents? Trends Microbiol 23:653–665

Perreau M, Pantaleo G, Kremer EJ (2008) Activation of a dendritic cell-T cell axis by Ad5 immune complexes creates an improved environment for replication of HIV in T cells. J Exp Med 205:2717–2725

Pincetic A, Bournazos S, DiLillo DJ, Maamary J, Wang TT, Dahan R, Fiebiger BM, Ravetch JV (2014) Type I and type II Fc receptors regulate innate and adaptive immunity. Nat Immunol 15:707–716

Pokric B, Sladic D, Juros S, Cajavec S (1993) Application of the immune complex for immune protection against viral disease. Vaccine 11:655–659

Polyanskaya N, Bergmeier LA, Sharpe SA, Cook N, Leech S, Hall G, Dennis M, ten Haaft P, Heeney J, Manca F, Lehner T, Cranage MP (2001) Mucosal exposure to subinfectious doses of SIV primes gut-associated antibody-secreting cells and T cells: lack of enhancement by nonneutralizing antibody. Virology 279:527–538

Qiao SW, Kobayashi K, Johansen FE, Sollid LM, Andersen JT, Milford E, Roopenian DC, Lencer WI, Blumberg RS (2008) Dependence of antibody-mediated presentation of antigen on FcRn. Proc Natl Acad Sci U S A 105:9337–9342

Rafiq K, Bergtold A, Clynes R (2002) Immune complex-mediated antigen presentation induces tumor immunity. J Clin Invest 110:71–79

Randall RE, Young DF (1988) Humoral and cytotoxic T cell immune responses to internal and external structural proteins of simian virus 5 induced by immunization with solid matrix-antibody-antigen complexes. J Gen Virol 69(Pt 10):2505–2516

Randall RE, Young DF (1991) Solid matrix-antibody-antigen complexes induce antigen-specific CD8+ cells that clear a persistent paramyxovirus infection. J Virol 65:719–726

Ravetch JV, Kinet JP (1991) Fc receptors. Annu Rev Immunol 9:457–492

Regnault A, Lankar D, Lacabanne V, Rodriguez A, Thery C, Rescigno M, Saito T, Verbeek S, Bonnerot C, Ricciardi-Castagnoli P, Amigorena S (1999) Fcgamma receptor-mediated induction of dendritic cell maturation and major histocompatibility complex class I-restricted antigen presentation after immune complex internalization. J Exp Med 189:371–380

Rock KL, Gamble S, Rothstein L (1990) Presentation of exogenous antigen with class I major histocompatibility complex molecules. Science 249:918–921

Sancho D, Mourao-Sa D, Joffre OP, Schulz O, Rogers NC, Pennington DJ, Carlyle JR, Reis e Sousa C (2008) Tumor therapy in mice via antigen targeting to a novel, DC-restricted C-type lectin. J Clin Invest 118:2098–2110

Savina A, Jancic C, Hugues S, Guermonprez P, Vargas P, Moura IC, Lennon-Dumenil AM, Seabra MC, Raposo G, Amigorena S (2006) NOX2 controls phagosomal pH to regulate antigen processing during crosspresentation by dendritic cells. Cell 126:205–218

Schat KA, da Silva Martins NR, O'Connell PH, Piepenbrink MS (2011) Immune complex vaccines for chicken infectious anemia virus. Avian Dis 55:90–96

Schmidt J, Blum HE, Thimme R (2013) T-cell responses in hepatitis B and C virus infection: similarities and differences. Emerg Microbes Infect 2:e15

Schuurhuis DH, Ioan-Facsinay A, Nagelkerken B, van Schip JJ, Sedlik C, Melief CJ, Verbeek JS, Ossendorp F (2002) Antigen-antibody immune complexes empower dendritic cells to efficiently prime specific CD8+ CTL responses in vivo. J Immunol 168:2240–2246

Seeger C, Mason WS (2015) Molecular biology of hepatitis B virus infection. Virology 0:672–686

Shiver JW, Emini EA (2004) Recent advances in the development of HIV-1 vaccines using replication-incompetent adenovirus vectors. Annu Rev Med 55:355–372

Simpson TR, Li F, Montalvo-Ortiz W, Sepulveda MA, Bergerhoff K, Arce F, Roddie C, Henry JY, Yagita H, Wolchok JD, Peggs KS, Ravetch JV, Allison JP, Quezada SA (2013) Fc-dependent depletion of tumor-infiltrating regulatory T cells co-defines the efficacy of anti-CTLA-4 therapy against melanoma. J Exp Med 210:1695–1710

St Pierre CA, Leonard D, Corvera S, Kurt-Jones EA, Finberg RW (2011) Antibodies to cell surface proteins redirect intracellular trafficking pathways. Exp Mol Pathol 91:723–732

Szakal AK, Kosco MH, Tew JG (1988a) FDC-iccosome mediated antigen delivery to germinal center B cells, antigen processing and presentation to T cells. Adv Exp Med Biol 237:197–202

Szakal AK, Kosco MH, Tew JG (1988b) A novel in vivo follicular dendritic cell-dependent iccosome-mediated mechanism for delivery of antigen to antigen-processing cells. J Immunol 140:341–353

Szecsi J, Gabriel G, Edfeldt G, Michelet M, Klenk HD, Cosset FL (2009) DNA vaccination with a single-plasmid construct coding for viruslike particles protects mice against infection with a highly pathogenic avian influenza A virus. J Infect Dis 200:181–190

Tao P, Luo M, Zhu D, Qu S, Yang Z, Gao M, Guo D, Pan Z (2009) Virus-like particle vaccine comprised of the HA, NA, and M1 proteins of an avian isolated H5N1 influenza virus induces protective immunity against homologous and heterologous strains in mice. Viral Immunol 22:273–281

Terres G, Wolins W (1959) Enhanced sensitization in mice by simultaneous injection of antigen and specific rabbit antiserum. Proc Soc Exp Biol Med 102:632–635

Terres G, Wolins W (1961) Enhanced immunological sensitization of mice by the simultaneous injection of antigen and specific antiserum. I. Effect of varying the amount of antigen used relative to the antiserum. J Immunol 86:361–368

Vasovic LV, Dyall R, Clynes RA, Ravetch JV, Nikolic-Zugic J (1997) Synergy between an antibody and CD8+ cells in eliminating an established tumor. Eur J Immunol 27:374–382

Visciano ML, Tuen M, Gorny MK, Hioe CE (2008) In vivo alteration of humoral responses to HIV-1 envelope glycoprotein gp120 by antibodies to the CD4-binding site of gp120. Virology 372:409–420

Walker LM, Phogat SK, Chan-Hui PY, Wagner D, Phung P, Goss JL, Wrin T, Simek MD, Fling S, Mitcham JL, Lehrman JK, Priddy FH, Olsen OA, Frey SM, Hammond PW, Protocol GPI, Kaminsky S, Zamb T, Moyle M, Koff WC, Poignard P, Burton DR (2009) Broad and potent neutralizing antibodies from an African donor reveal a new HIV-1 vaccine target. Science 326:285–289

Wang TT, Maamary J, Tan GS, Bournazos S, Davis CW, Krammer F, Schlesinger SJ, Palese P, Ahmed R, Ravetch JV (2015) Anti-HA glycoforms drive B cell affinity selection and determine influenza vaccine efficacy. Cell 162:160–169

Wang W, Sun L, Li T, Ma Y, Li J, Liu Y, Li M, Wang L, Li C, Xie Y, Wen Y, Liang M, Chen L, Tong S (2016) A human monoclonal antibody against small envelope protein of hepatitis B virus with potent neutralization effect. MAbs 8:468–477

Wen Y, Shi Y (2016) Alum: an old dog with new tricks. Emerg Microbes Infect 5:e25

Wen YM (2009) Antigen-antibody immunogenic complex: promising novel vaccines for microbial persistent infections. Expert Opin Biol Ther 9:285–291

Wen YM, Wu XH, Hu DC, Zhang QP, Guo SQ (1995) Hepatitis B vaccine and anti-HBs complex as approach for vaccine therapy. Lancet 345:1575–1576

Wen YM, Xiong SD, Zhang W (1994) Solid matrix-antibody-antigen complex can clear viraemia and antigenaemia in persistent duck hepatitis B virus infection. J Gen Virol 75(Pt 2):335–339

Wieland A, Shashidharamurthy R, Kamphorst AO, Han JH, Aubert RD, Choudhury BP, Stowell SR, Lee J, Punkosdy GA, Shlomchik MJ, Selvaraj P, Ahmed R (2015) Antibody effector functions mediated by Fcgamma-receptors are compromised during persistent viral infection. Immunity 42:367–378

Wolpoe ME, Lutz ER, Ercolini AM, Murata S, Ivie SE, Garrett ES, Emens LA, Jaffee EM, Reilly RT (2003) HER-2/neu-specific monoclonal antibodies collaborate with HER-2/neu-targeted granulocyte macrophage colony-stimulating factor secreting whole cell vaccination to augment CD8+ T cell effector function and tumor-free survival in Her-2/neu-transgenic mice. J Immunol 171:2161–2169

Wu X, Yang ZY, Li Y, Hogerkorp CM, Schief WR, Seaman MS, Zhou T, Schmidt SD, Wu L, Xu L, Longo NS, McKee K, O'Dell S, Louder MK, Wycuff DL, Feng Y, Nason M, Doria-Rose N, Connors M, Kwong PD, Roederer M, Wyatt RT, Nabel GJ, Mascola JR (2010) Rational design of envelope identifies broadly neutralizing human monoclonal antibodies to HIV-1. Science 329:856–861

Wu Y, Sukumar S, El Shikh ME, Best AM, Szakal AK, Tew JG (2008) Immune complex-bearing follicular dendritic cells deliver a late antigenic signal that promotes somatic hypermutation. J Immunol 180:281–290

Xu DZ, Huang KL, Zhao K, Xu LF, Shi N, Yuan ZH, Wen YM (2005) Vaccination with recombinant HBsAg-HBIG complex in healthy adults. Vaccine 23:2658–2664

Yamada DH, Elsaesser H, Lux A, Timmerman JM, Morrison SL, de la Torre JC, Nimmerjahn F, Brooks DG (2015) Suppression of Fcgamma-receptor-mediated antibody effector function during persistent viral infection. Immunity 42:379–390

Yao X, Zheng B, Zhou J, Xu DZ, Zhao K, Sun SH, Yuan ZH, Wen YM (2007) Therapeutic effect of hepatitis B surface antigen-antibody complex is associated with cytolytic and non-cytolytic immune responses in hepatitis B patients. Vaccine 25:1771–1779

Yoshida M, Claypool SM, Wagner JS, Mizoguchi E, Mizoguchi A, Roopenian DC, Lencer WI, Blumberg RS (2004) Human neonatal Fc receptor mediates transport of IgG into luminal secretions for delivery of antigens to mucosal dendritic cells. Immunity 20:769–783

Zhang TY, Yuan Q, Zhao JH, Zhang YL, Yuan LZ, Lan Y, Lo YC, Sun CP, Wu CR, Zhang JF, Zhang Y, Cao JL, Guo XR, Liu X, Mo XB, Luo WX, Cheng T, Chen YX, Tao MH, Shih JW, Zhao QJ, Zhang J, Chen PJ, Yuan YA, Xia NS (2016) Prolonged suppression of HBV in mice by a novel antibody that targets a unique epitope on hepatitis B surface antigen. Gut 65:658–671

Zheng B, Zhang Y, He H, Marinova E, Switzer K, Wansley D, Mbawuike I, Han S (2007) Rectification of age-associated deficiency in cytotoxic T cell response to influenza A virus by immunization with immune complexes. J Immunol 179:6153–6159

Zheng BJ, Ng MH, He LF, Yao X, Chan KW, Yuen KY, Wen YM (2001) Therapeutic efficacy of hepatitis B surface antigen-antibodies-recombinant DNA composite in HBsAg transgenic mice. Vaccine 19:4219–4225

Zhou C, Li C, Gong GZ, Wang S, Zhang JM, Xu DZ, Guo LM, Ren H, Xu M, Xie Q, Pan C, Xu J, Hu Z, Geng S, Zhou X, Wang X, Zhou X, Mi H, Zhao G, Yu W, Wen YM, Huang L, Wang XY, Wang B (2017) Analysis of immunological mechanisms exerted by HBsAg-HBIG therapeutic vaccine combined with Adefovir in chronic hepatitis B patients. Hum Vaccin Immunother 13:1989–1996

Fc Receptors in Antimicrobial Protection

Andreas Wieland and Rafi Ahmed

Contents

Abstract Antibodies are the key effector molecules of the humoral immune system providing long-term protective immunity against a wide range of pathogens and regulating immune responses. Traditionally, antibody-mediated protection against microbes was thought to be mainly a result of neutralizing Fab–antigen interaction; however, an increasing number of studies show the importance of proper FcR engagement for the protective capacity of antimicrobial antibodies. In this chapter, we review FcR-mediated effector functions contributing to antimicrobial protection in a direct and indirect manner. Furthermore, we highlight recent findings about the important role of Fc–FcR interactions for antimicrobial protection in vivo and provide examples demonstrating the crucial role of proper FcR engagement for antibody-mediated protection against viruses, bacteria, fungi, and parasites.

A. Wieland (✉) · R. Ahmed
Department of Microbiology & Immunology, School of Medicine,
Emory University, 1510 Clifton Road, Atlanta, GA, USA
e-mail: andreas.wieland@emory.edu

Current Topics in Microbiology and Immunology (2019) 423: 119–150
https://doi.org/10.1007/82_2019_154
Published online: 22 February 2019

1   Introduction

Antibodies are involved in the protection against a wide range of pathogens including viruses, bacteria, fungi, and parasites and are the correlate of protection for the vast majority of available vaccines (Plotkin 2010). Vaccination and/or infection can induce the generation of long-lived plasma cells residing mainly in the bone marrow and producing high quantities of pathogen-specific antibodies conferring long-term protective immunity (Manz et al. 1997; Slifka et al. 1998). The ability to mount an antibody response against an almost unlimited number of target structures and generate highly specific antibodies is accomplished through somatic recombination and hypermutation of the Fab (fragment, antibody binding) domain. While the variable Fab domain mediates antigen specificity and binds its respective antigen, the Fc (fragment, crystallizable) domain can engage FcRs expressed on leukocytes to mediated diverse effector functions. The interactions between the Fc domain of IgG and FcγRs as well as the resulting cellular effector functions are well defined (Bournazos et al. 2017). Although the Fc domain of IgG is traditionally considered to be an invariable region, the existence of different IgG subclasses with divergent amino acid sequences and the differential composition of the bianntennary N-linked glycan at the conserved glycosylation site Asn297 results in substantial heterogeneity in this region. This structural heterogeneity affects the capacity of the Fc domain to interact with type I and type II FcγRs and subsequently modulates the effector functions elicited by IgG (Bournazos et al. 2017).

FcγRs are expressed by different leukocytes of the myeloid and lymphoid lineage, both in circulation as well as in tissues, and thus FcγR-signaling can modulate several immunological processes besides direct cytotoxic IgG-mediated effector functions such as phagocytosis and cellular cytotoxicity (Pincetic et al. 2014). Different leukocyte populations are characterized by distinct FcγR expression patterns and FcγR expression levels are a function of cellular differentiation, cell activation status as well as environmental cues (inflammation, infection, injury) allowing to further modulate FcγR-mediated effector functions in a context-dependent manner (te Velde et al. 1992; Uciechowski et al. 1998; Anthony et al. 2011; Dugast et al. 2011; Smith et al. 2012; Pincetic et al. 2014). While all IgG-mediated cytotoxic effector functions critically depend on the engagement of activating type I FcγRs, the balanced engagement of activating and inhibitory type I Fcγs as well as type II FcγRs by IgG can affect a wide range of immunological processes involved in antimicrobial immunity, ranging from antigen uptake and presentation, differentiation and activation of antigen-presenting cells, secretion of cytokines and chemokines, modulation of T cell activation, affinity maturation of B cells and plasma cell survival (Bournazos and Ravetch 2015).

Antibodies are the correlate of protection for the vast majority of available vaccines and various in vitro assays such as toxin/virus neutralization, bactericidal assay, and opsonophagocytosis are employed to quantify pathogen-specific antibody responses correlated with protection (Plotkin 2010). However, several studies demonstrated that Fc–FcγR interactions play an important role in the protective capacity of neutralizing antibodies against various pathogens and toxins in vivo that cannot be predicted by simple in vitro experiments (Abboud et al. 2010; Bournazos et al. 2014a; DiLillo et al. 2014; Hessell et al. 2007). These observations sparked an enormous interest in elucidating the contributions of in vivo Fc–FcγR interactions in antimicrobial protection with the ultimate goal to further enhance FcR-mediated antimicrobial effector functions of antibody-based therapeutics.

Here, we review FcR-mediated effector functions contributing to antimicrobial protection, highlight the important role of Fc–FcR interactions for antimicrobial protection in vivo, and briefly discuss microbial evasion strategies. Our review focusses on the role of FcγRs as its ligand IgG is by far the most prevalent isotype in the serum and the role of FcγRs in antimicrobial protection has been extensively studied.

2 FcR-Mediated Effector Functions with Direct Antimicrobial Activity

2.1 Antibody-Dependent Phagocytosis

Phagocytosis, first observed over 100 years ago, is a critical component of the immune system capable of integrating both innate and adaptive immune responses to combat pathogens. Although phagocytosis is traditionally defined as the cellular ingestion of large ($\geq$ 0.5-μm) particles (Flannagan et al. 2012), we use the term phagocytosis in the following indiscriminately of particle size. The engagement of type I FcγRs on phagocytic cells such as macrophages and neutrophils results in the efficient phagocytosis of IgG-opsonized particles that can range in size from single molecules, microbial pathogens to intact infected cells (Fig. 1). Although the phagocytic capacity varies among different phagocytes and might also be influenced by activation status and metabolic state of a cell (Pavlou et al. 2017), the downstream signaling cascade and mechanisms induced by FcγR cross-linking on the cell surface is common to all leukocytes expressing activating type I FcγRs.

The process of antibody-dependent cellular phagocytosis (ADCP) of IgG-opsonized particles by FcγRs can be subdivided into three distinct steps: (i) binding of IgG-opsonized particles to FcγRs on the cell surface of phagocytes, (ii) clustering and oligomerization of FcγRs, inducing a signaling cascade; followed by (iii) engulfment of the opsonized particle by an actin-driven process (Flannagan et al. 2012). The successful phagocytic uptake of an IgG-opsonized particle is an iterative process that requires, in addition to the initial attachment event, circumferential engagement of unoccupied FcγRs by particle-bound IgG (Griffin et al. 1975). The circumferential interaction between membrane-bound FcγRs and IgG on the particle is thought to guide the pseudopod extensions as the phagocyte membrane slowly zippers around the particle.

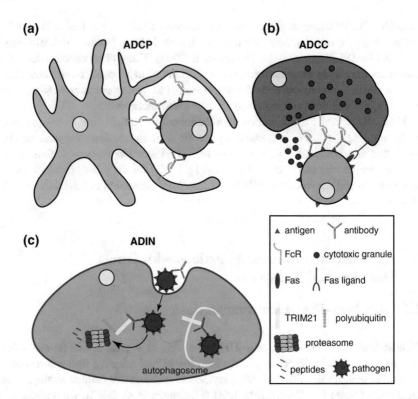

Fig. 1 FcR-mediated antibody effector functions with direct antimicrobial activity. **a** Antibody-dependent cellular phagocytosis (ADCP). **b** Antibody-dependent cellular cytotoxicity (ADCC). **c** Antibody-dependent intracellular neutralization (ADIN)

The binding of immune complexes to activating type I FcγRs results in clustering of the receptors on the cell surface followed by the phosphorylation of the intracellular immunoreceptor tyrosine-based activation motif (ITAM) domain by tyrosine kinases of the Src family including Lyn, Lck, Hck, and Fgr (Hamada et al. 1993; Durden et al. 1995; Pignata et al. 1993; Jouvin et al. 1994). Following the phosphorylation of both tyrosines of the ITAM, the recruitment and activation of Syk is essential for FcγR-mediated phagocytosis as in the absence of Syk phagocytic cup formation is initiated but arrested early on (Crowley et al. 1997; Kiefer et al. 1998). ITAM phosphorylation also results in the activation of ζ-chain subunits, ZAP70, and FAK regulating actin polymerization, phagocytosis and actin polymerization (Jouvin et al. 1994; Swanson and Hoppe 2004; Hamawy et al. 1995). Phosphorylation of Syk leads to a recruitment cascade of several signaling adaptor proteins to the activated FcγR complex (Flannagan et al. 2012). Syk and additionally recruited adaptor proteins subsequently induce activation of class I phosphatidylinositol 3-kinase (PI3K) and phospholipase C γ (PLCγ), which generates the metabolites diacylglyercol (DAG), an efficient activator of protein kinase C (PKC), and inositol-triphosphate (IP3) (Liao et al. 1992; Kanakaraj et al. 1994;

Ninomiya et al. 1994). The above-mentioned signaling processes seem to contribute to efficient phagocytosis in distinct ways as PKCε recruitment can enhance phagocytosis independently of actin polymerization and PI3K activity seems to be essential for the phagocytosis of large ($\geq$ 3-μm) particles by promoting maximal pseudopod extension, but only has a minimal impact on the phagocytosis of smaller particles (Larsen et al. 2002; Araki et al. 1996; Cox et al. 1999). In addition, the activation of the PI3K-PKC pathway also results in intracellular Ca^{2+} mobilization from the endoplasmatic reticulum and cellular activation (Bournazos and Ravetch 2015; Odin et al. 1991). Further, signaling proteins involved in FcγR-mediated phagocytosis encompass several GTPases of the Rho family such as Cdc42, Rac1, and Rac2, which are key regulators of actin polymerization and remodeling (Hoppe and Swanson 2004; Caron and Hall 1998; Park and Cox 2009). These GTPases modulate the activity of the Arp2/3 nucleator complex, which supports actin polymerization upon FcγR signaling, through additional mediator proteins such as Wiskott-Aldrich syndrome protein (May et al. 2000; Lorenzi et al. 2000).

The signaling cascade induced by the engagement of activating type I FcγRs is counterbalanced by the engagement of the inhibitory type I FcγR, FcγRIIb, and thus FcγR-mediated effector functions such as phagocytosis are a result of the cumulative signaling from activating and inhibitory type I FcγRs (Nimmerjahn and Ravetch 2005). FcγRIIb contains a single-tyrosine signaling domain known as immunoreceptor tyrosine-based inhibition motif (ITIM). Following receptor clustering and phosphorylation by kinases of the Src family, the ITIM of FcγRIIb recruits several phosphatases like SHIP, SHP-1, and SHP-2 (Pearse et al. 1999; Amigorena et al. 1992a, Muta et al. 1994). SHIP is an inositol 5-phosphatase and inhibits phagocytosis by hydrolysis of phosphatidylinositol 3,4,5-triphosphate thus inhibiting the recruitment and activation of PLCγ and BTK (Bournazos and Ravetch 2015). SHP-1, a phosphotyrosine-specific protein phosphatase, has been shown to inhibit FcγR-mediated phagocytosis through a mechanism involving the ubiquitin ligase Cbl (Kant et al. 2002). SHIP and SHP-1 have also been shown to associate with the monophosphorylated ITAM of FcγRs, suggesting a built-in regulatory feedback of stimulatory receptors (Nakamura et al. 2002; Ganesan et al. 2003). The balanced signaling through activating and inhibitory FcγRs is thus supposed to ensure optimal effector activity and, at the same time, prevent excessive pathogenic immune activation (Bournazos et al. 2017). Phagocytic activity directed against pathogen-infected host cells can be further regulated by the engagement of various inhibitory receptors expressed on phagocytes such as Siglec-5, Siglec-9, and signal-regulating protein (SIRP)-α (Steevels and Meyaard 2011). The interaction of SIRP-α with its ubiquitously expressed ligand CD47, which is commonly referred to as a "do not eat me signal" or "marker of self," is well studied and shown to increase the activation threshold required for efficient FcγR-mediated phagocytosis of host cells by activation of SHP-1 (Oldenborg et al. 2001; Okazawa et al. 2005).

The successful internalization of opsonized particles results in the formation of a phagosome, which in its initial immature state is unable to mediate the destruction of the engulfed pathogen. However, through sequential highly orchestrated membrane fusion and fission events, termed phagosome maturation, the composition of the phagosome changes dramatically in order to be equipped with the necessary tools to destroy the engulfed pathogen (Desjardins et al. 1994). The sequential fusion of the phagosome with discrete endosomal compartments results in a stepwise acidification of the lumen. The mature phagosome/phagolysosome generated by the fusion of late phagosomes with lysosomes is a highly microbicidal organelle characterized by a highly acidic (pH $\approx$4.5) and oxidative environment due to reactive oxygen species (ROS) (Flannagan et al. 2012). Furthermore, mature phagosomes also contain an arsenal of antimicrobial peptides and more than 50 different hydrolytic enzymes such as lysozyme and cathepsins to ensure complete digestion of complex pathogens.

2.2 Antibody-Dependent Cellular Cytotoxicity

Antibody-dependent cellular cytotoxicity (ADCC) was first described about 50 years ago as the ability of nonimmune lymphoid cells—now known as natural killer (NK) cells—to efficiently lyse antibody-coated target cells in vitro (Moller 1967). The expression of FcRs on the surface of cytotoxic effector cells is a requirement for ADCC and multiple activating FcRs have been shown to mediate ADCC upon binding to antibody-coated target cells and subsequent cross-linking of FcRs. In humans, engagement of all activating type I FcγRs (FcγRI, FcγRIIa/c, and FcγRIIIa) as well as the IgA-binding FcαRI (CD89) and the IgE-binding FcϵRI can trigger ADCC (Bournazos et al. 2017; Morton et al. 1996; Fu et al. 2008). Whereas the intracellular signals transduced upon cross-linking of activating type I FcγRs are common to all leukocytes expressing activating type I FcγRs (described in 2.1), the interpretation of these signals and thus the resulting biological response (i.e., ADCC, ADCP, cytokine secretion, …) varies among different leukocyte subsets (Bournazos et al. 2017), probably representing a function of cell-type-specific commitment and modulating environmental cues. ADCC represents a mechanism complementary to ADCP that can mediate the destruction of pathogens exceeding the size limitations of phagocytosis or of infected cells that cannot be readily phagocytosed.

The main cytotoxic effector populations capable of ADCC include NK cells, neutrophils, and eosinophils. NK cells are most studied effectors of ADCC and freshly isolated NK cells exhibit efficient ADCC toward antibody-coated target cells in vitro. NK cells express relatively high levels of FcγRIIIa at steady state and are the only leukocyte population expressing only an activating type I FcγR but not the inhibitory FcγRIIb (Bournazos et al. 2017). However, NK cells can express several inhibitory receptors such as killer Ig-like receptors (KIRs), CD94-NKG2, and immunoglobulin-like receptor (LIR), which can counterbalance FcγRIIIa activation via SHP-1 and SHP-2 (Pegram et al. 2011). Circulating neutrophils expressing FcγRIIa, FcγRIIb, and FcγRIIIb, exhibit limited cytotoxic potential in their normal resting state, but can be activated by several cytokines such as granulocyte-macrophage colony-stimulating factor (GM-CSF) and granulocyte colony-stimulating factor (G-CSF) (Bournazos et al. 2017; Kato and Kitagawa 2006). Interferon (IFN)γ signaling can further induce FcγRI expression on neutrophils. Furthermore, neutrophils express FcαRI endowing them with the ability to lyse IgA-coated target cells (Otten et al. 2005). Eosinophils express FcγRIIa and FcγRIIb at a resting state and upregulate expression of FcγRI and FcγRIIIb upon cytokine stimulation. Like neutrophils, eosinophils require cytokine-mediated activation prior to exerting efficient degranulation (Fabian et al. 1992). In addition to responding to IgG-coated targets, eosinophils can also exert potent cytolytic activity against IgA- and IgE-coated targets through FcαRI and FcεRI (Abu-Ghazaleh et al. 1989; Dombrowicz et al. 2000).

The exact processes involved in ADCC have been best studied in NK cells and share many similarities with cytotoxic T cells. Upon FcR-mediated activation, effector cells release specialized granules at the lytic synapse by a calcium-dependent polarized exocytotic process (de Saint Basile et al. 2010). The composition of these lytic granules varies considerably between NK cells and granulocytes and even between various granulocyte subsets. NK cells are well equipped to lyse pathogen-infected host cells using granules containing the pore-forming protein perforin and granzyme B, a serine protease which induces apoptosis upon entry into the target cell and activation of caspase (Voskoboinik et al. 2015). In addition to lysis of infected host cells, NK cells also seem to be able to directly kill bacteria by the release of perforin and granulysin (Lu et al. 2014). Upon FcγR engagement, NK cells upregulate Fas ligand enabling them to kill target cells expressing Fas through a granule-independent mechanism (Fig. 1) (Eischen et al. 1996). The granules of granulocytes contain a cell-type- and activation-state-specific mixture of preformed effector molecules and are released upon FcγR engagement (Jonsson et al. 2013). These granules typically contain proteases (elastase, cathepsins, collagenase), antimicrobial peptides and proteins (defensins, cathelicidins, lysozyme, lactoferrin), enzymes (peroxidase, alkaline phosphatase), and leukotrienes which mediate inflammation and recruitment of additional leukocytes (Bournazos et al. 2016). FcγR signaling in granulocytes also results in the generation of reactive oxygen intermediates (ROI) through the formation and activation of the NADPH-dependent oxidase complex (Suh et al. 2006). This results in the production of superoxide anions exhibiting direct cytotoxic activity and serving as reactive intermediates to generate a plethora of reactive oxygen species such as hydrogen peroxide (H_2O_2), hydroxyl radical (OH·), and hypochlorous acid (HOCl)(Nathan and Cunningham-Bussel 2013).

Although NK-cell-mediated ADCC of antibody-coated target cells has been extensively studied in vitro, the exact contribution of NK-cell-mediated ADCC to antimicrobial protection in vivo is less defined due to the overwhelming contribution of phagocytic active cells to antibody-mediated protection in vivo. Future studies employing sophisticated depletion strategies and/or genetic knockout models will be able to address the exact role of the various cell populations capable of ADCC for antimicrobial protection in vivo.

2.3   Antibody-Dependent Intracellular Neutralization

The term antibody-dependent intracellular neutralization (ADIN) was coined to describe antibody effector mechanisms mediated through the cytosolic Fc receptor tripartite motif 21 (TRIM21). TRIM21, an IFN-inducible member of the TRIM protein family of RING E3 ubiquitin ligases, is a broadly expressed cytosolic Fc receptor that is widely conserved among mammals and structurally unrelated to other classes of Fc receptors (James et al. 2007; Keeble et al. 2008; Reymond et al. 2001). TRIM21 interacts with the C_H2-C_H3 domain interface of the IgG Fc and is unique in its ability to bind with high affinity to all IgG isotypes as well as, although with lower affinity, to IgA and IgM (Mallery et al. 2010; Bidgood et al. 2014).

Pathogens such as non-enveloped viruses, that have entered the cytosol of a cell and have antibodies bound to their capsid, can be recognized by TRIM21 (Mallery et al. 2010; Bidgood et al. 2014). TRIM21 engagement results in autoubiquitination mediated by the E3 activity of the RING domain and the subsequent recruitment of the proteasomal machinery (Fig. 1) (Mallery et al. 2010). Due to size constraints of the proteasomal barrel, TRIM21-degradation of viral particles by the proteasome requires the additional recruitment of the AAA ATPase v97/VCP, which is capable of extracting proteins from larger complexes and unfolding them (Hauler et al. 2012). TRIM21 has also been suggested to trigger autophagy to protect from intracellular opsonized bacteria, which have been shown to colocalize with the autophagosomal marker LC3 (Rakebrandt et al. 2014). In general, ADIN-mediated protection has been shown to be a function of TRIM21 expression and the extent of opsonization with the expression level of TRIM21 being the dominant determinant (McEwan et al. 2012). ADIN can thus provide a last line of defense in case neutralizing antibodies were not abundant enough to completely block pathogen entry and classical FcR-mediated antibody effector functions were insufficient or evaded by the pathogen. However, as ADIN has been mainly studied in vitro, its role in pathogen control in vivo has not been addressed in detail.

In addition to ADIN, the recognition of cytosolic immunoglobulins by TRIM21 induces the activation of innate signaling pathways, resulting in the production of several pro-inflammatory cytokines and chemokines mediating an antiviral state which could potentially further upregulate TRIM21 in neighboring cells (McEwan et al. 2013).

3   FcR-Mediated Effector Functions Contributing to Antimicrobial Protection

The engagement of FcRs not only triggers direct effector mechanisms resulting in pathogen clearance, but is also involved in the regulation of several immunological processes ultimately contributing to antimicrobial protection (Fig. 2). In this section, we briefly discuss the role of FcRs in modulating immunological processes involved in antimicrobial protection.

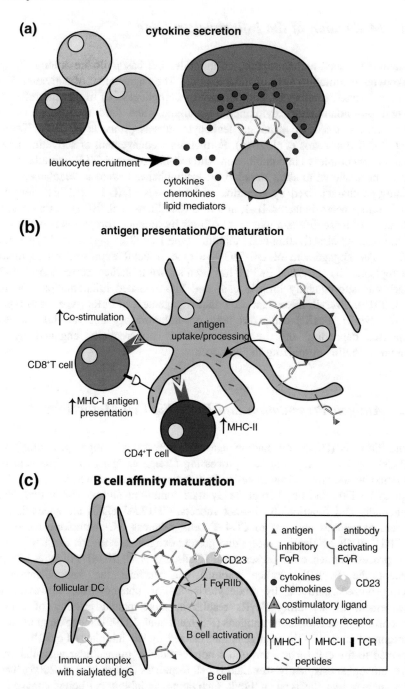

Fig. 2 FcR-mediated antibody effector functions indirectly contributing to antimicrobial protection. **a** Cytokine secretion. **b** Antigen presentation and maturation of dendritic cells (DC). **c** B cell affinity maturation

3.1 Modulation of the Inflammatory State

Granulocytes such as neutrophils, eosinophils, and basophils are among the first leukocytes recruited to sites of inflammation. The engagement of activating FcRs on granulocytes, monocytes, and polarized macrophages can trigger the release of several pro-inflammatory cytokines, chemokines, and lipid mediators that will result in recruitment of additional leukocyte subsets (Stone et al. 2010; Tecchio et al. 2014; Bournazos et al. 2016). Furthermore, engagement of activating FcγRs by immune complexes in combination with toll-like receptor (TLR) stimulation has further been shown to skew unpolarized macrophages toward a "regulatory" M2b phenotype characterized by secretion of low levels of IL-12 and high levels of IL-10, tumor necrosis factor, IL-1, and IL-6 (Guilliams et al. 2014). Ultimately, the activation of these different leukocyte subsets by immune complexes is determined by the balance of activating and inhibitory type I FcγR engagement (Clynes et al. 1999). The engagement of DC-SIGN, a type II FcγR expressed on regulatory macrophages, by sialylated IgG Fc has been shown to induce expression of IL-33, which can subsequently limit T cell- and IgG-mediated inflammation (Fiebiger et al. 2015). Overall, these data show that engagement of FcRs (type I and type II FcγRs, FcαRI, FcεRI) can exert both pro-inflammatory and anti-inflammatory responses depending on the types of FcRs preferentially engaged by the immunoglobulins opsonizing the pathogen.

3.2 Antigen Presentation and Dendritic Cell Maturation

Dendritic cells (DCs) and macrophages are professional antigen-presenting cells (APCs) capable of ingesting and processing foreign antigens for subsequent presentation to adaptive immune cells. Conventional human dendritic cells (cDCs) express FcγRIIa and FcγRIIb at steady-state conditions and consist of two developmentally and functionally distinct subsets: $CD172\alpha^+$ cDCs are specialized to present exogenous antigens to CD4 T cells, whereas XC-chemokine receptor 1 $(XCR1)^+$ cDCs efficiently process and present exogenous antigens to $CD8^+$ T cells in a process termed cross-presentation (Guilliams et al. 2014). All type I FcγRs (except the FcγRIIb1 splice variant) can mediate the internalization of IgG-opsonized particles by endocytosis and/or phagocytosis; however, the engagement of activating FcγRs results in more potent priming of cellular responses against exogenous antigens (Regnault et al. 1999; Dhodapkar et al. 2002; Amigorena et al. 1992b). Antigens internalized by the inhibitory FcγRIIb can be recycled to the cell surface through a nondegradative intracellular vesicular compartment and subsequently stimulate B cell responses (Bergtold et al. 2005). These data suggest that the type of FcγR (activating or inhibitory) being engaged by IgG-opsonized antigen influences the degradation pathway the antigen will be subjected to and, ultimately, the kind of immune response being stimulated.

The engagement of activating type I FcγRs on DCs by immune complexes does not only mediate efficient antigen uptake and subsequent antigen presentation on MHC class I and MHC class II molecules, but also triggers a pro-inflammatory signaling cascade resulting in DC maturation, which is characterized by increased expression of MHC and co-stimulatory molecules such as CD80 and CD86 as well as overall enhanced antigen presentation and is required for the efficient induction of effector responses (Guilliams et al. 2014). Engagement of FcγRs on DCs by immune complexes alone is not sufficient to induce DC maturation and effector T cell responses, as DCs express both inhibitory as well as activating type I FcγRs and signaling through activating type I FcγRs is counteracted by the inhibitory FcγRIIb in DCs, like in other leukocyte populations. DC maturation in response to immune complexes thus requires additional co-stimulatory signals to overcome the inhibitory signaling through FcγRIIb, which can be provided by engagement of TLRs (Bournazos et al. 2016). The amount of additional co-stimulation required for DC maturation in response to immune complexes depends on the amount of signaling received through activating FcγRs relative to inhibitory FcγRIIb, which is determined by the expression levels of activating and inhibitory type I FcγRs. FcγR expression on DCs can be dramatically altered based on the local inflammatory milieu with IFNγ inducing expression of FcγRI and downregulation of FcγRIIb, and IL-4 increasing FcγRIIb expression (Pricop et al. 2001; Uciechowski et al. 1998; Boruchov et al. 2005). DCs can thus integrate signals from the local inflammatory milieu to adjust the threshold required for IgG-mediated maturation. Overall, these studies demonstrate that FcγRs play an important role in the induction of cellular immune responses to opsonized antigens by regulating antigen uptake, presentation as well as maturation.

3.3   B Cell Selection and Affinity Maturation

B cells are the sole leukocyte population that constitutively expresses the inhibitory FcγRIIb but lacks expression of any activating type I FcγR. In addition, B cells also express the type II FcγR CD23, which was initially identified as low-affinity FcR for IgE and recently shown to bind sialylated IgG-containing immune complexes (Sondermann et al. 2013). The role of inhibitory signaling through FcγRIIb in B cells and its role during B cell selection is well defined. Engagement of FcγRIIb without concomitant B cell receptor (BCR) engagement induces proapoptotic signals, which are attenuated upon co-aggregation with BCR resulting in B cell survival (Ono et al. 1997; Pearse et al. 1999). In the presence of IgG-complexed antigen, this mechanism thus allows for the selective survival of B cells with high affinity for the antigen, whereas nonspecific and low-affinity B cells are more likely to undergo apoptosis. The expression of FcγRIIb on B cells also sets an elevated activation threshold for effective BCR engagement by IgG-containing immune complexes and allows the generation of high-affinity antibody responses, while preventing the induction of low-affinity and potentially auto-reactive antibody responses (Ono et al. 1996, 1997; Pearse et al. 1999; Bolland and Ravetch 2000; Bolland et al. 2002). FcγRIIb expression on follicular DCs further supports the affinity maturation of B cells by promoting the retention of IgG-complexes in germinal centers (Qin et al. 2000).

Binding of the type II FcγR CD23 to sialylated IgG immune complexes has recently been shown to drive the generation of high-affinity IgG responses with broadly neutralizing capacity (Wang et al. 2015). The binding of sialylated IgG immune complexes to CD23 on B cells induced the upregulation of FcγRIIb, which in turn elevated the threshold required for B cell activation and resulted in the selection of high-affinity B cell clones. Overall, these studies demonstrate that both type I and type II FcγRs play an important role in regulating the humoral immune response and inducing effective antimicrobial antibody responses.

4 The Role of FcRs in Antimicrobial Protection

Antibodies are the correlate of protection against a wide range of pathogens and neutralizing antibodies can confer sterilizing immunity (Plotkin 2010). However, commonly used in vitro assays to assess the protective capacity of antibodies such as in vitro neutralization assays cannot efficiently predict their protective capacity in vivo as they fail to account for FcR-mediated effector functions carried out by various immune cell subsets. In this section, we highlight several studies demonstrating the crucial role of Fc–FcR interactions for in vivo protection and provide selected examples of FcR-dependent protection against viruses, bacteria, fungi, and parasites.

4.1 Viruses

4.1.1 Influenza

Neutralizing antibodies against influenza viruses, especially against the hemagglutinin (HA) protein which mediates viral attachment and fusion, are considered the main correlate of protection (Plotkin 2010). Neutralizing HA-specific antibodies can be directed against the head region surrounding the receptor-binding site of HA and thereby prevent viral attachment to sialic acid on target cells, or against the stalk of HA blocking viral fusion with the target cells (Ekiert et al. 2009). The globular head of HA is highly variable and most neutralizing head-reactive antibodies are strain-specific. In contrast, the HA stalk is relatively conserved and stalk-specific antibodies are broadly neutralizing influenza viruses across several strains and even subtypes (Wrammert et al. 2011; Corti et al. 2011).

Several studies have recently addressed the role of Fc–FcγR interactions for the in vivo protective capacity of mAbs directed against the head and stalk of HA

(Corti et al. 2011; DiLillo et al. 2014, 2016). While head-reactive neutralizing antibodies were protective at low doses and independent of FcγR engagement, stalk-reactive broadly neutralizing antibodies (bnAbs) required FcγR interactions to provide optimal protection or high concentrations for partial protection in vivo (DiLillo et al. 2014). Although bnAbs exhibit in vitro neutralizing activity, significantly higher concentrations of bnAbs (10–1000-fold) are required to achieve in vitro neutralization comparable to strain-specific antibodies (DiLillo et al. 2016). The engagement of activating type I FcγRs in vivo can, however, efficiently compensate for the inferior in vitro neutralization activity. The engagement of FcγRs on NK cells by bnAbs but not head-specific antibodies bound to influenza-infected target cells induces ADCC in vitro, suggesting that bnAbs mediate efficient in vivo protection by triggering ADCC/ADCP in vivo (Corti et al. 2011; DiLillo et al. 2014). Furthermore, a comprehensive comparison of 13 HA-specific mAbs including strain-specific neutralizing mAbs, bnAbs against the head and stalk of HA as well as head-reactive but not neutralizing mAbs revealed that all broadly reactive HA-specific antibodies require the engagement of activating type I FcγRs to mediate protection in vivo (DiLillo et al. 2016). It is not well understood why strain-specific and broadly reactive HA mAbs differ in their ability to induce FcγR-mediated effector functions. Reduced antigen affinity has been suggested to increase FcγR engagement by favoring monovalent antibody–antigen interactions resulting in a more densely opsonized target (Mazor et al. 2016). Furthermore, a recent study also demonstrated that, in addition to FcγR engagement, FcγR-mediated ADCC also required the receptor-binding domain of HA to bind with sialic acid on the effector cells (Leon et al. 2016), thus providing an explanation why neutralizing antibodies directed against the receptor-binding domain do not efficiently mediate FcγR-mediated effector functions.

Although most influenza studies focus on antibodies directed against HA due to its abundance on the viral particle and the fact that HA inhibition titers of $\geq 1:40$ are a correlate of protection, antibodies directed against neuraminidase (NA), and the matrix protein 2 (M2) can also provide protection from lethal influenza challenge in vivo (El Bakkouri et al. 2011; DiLillo et al. 2016; Memoli et al. 2016). Antibodies directed against M2 are not neutralizing and solely depend on the engagement of activating type I FcγRs for in vivo protection, which is mediated by alveolar macrophages through ADCC/ADCP (El Bakkouri et al. 2011). Although neutralizing NA-specific antibodies cannot prevent the initial infection, they can efficiently prevent viral budding and spread. Interestingly, in accordance with results obtained for HA-specific bnAbs and their reduced in vitro neutralization capability, bnAbs against NA but not strain-specific NA antibodies required FcγR engagement for in vivo protection (DiLillo et al. 2016). Overall, these results demonstrate that neutralizing antibodies with inferior in vitro activity can confer superior protection in vivo if they can efficiently engage FcγRs.

4.1.2 Human Immunodeficiency Virus

The envelope glycoprotein (env) of human immunodeficiency virus (HIV) is the major target for the development of neutralizing antibodies against HIV, and several bnAbs have been developed despite its sequence diversity, glycan shield and low abundance on the viral particle. Fc–FcγR interactions play an important role during HIV infection as patients homozygous for the low-affinity variant of FcγRIIa progress faster to AIDS (Forthal et al. 2007). BnAbs against HIV require the efficient engagement of FcγRs to provide in vivo protection as a bnAb unable to efficiently engage FcγRs failed to provide in vivo protection against SHIV challenge in nonhuman primates (Hessell et al. 2007). Mechanistic studies of several bnAbs in mouse models subsequently showed that the engagement of activating type I FcγRs and triggering of FcγR-mediated effector functions substantially contributed to their capacity to block viral entry and suppress viremia (Bournazos et al. 2014b). Furthermore, Fc–FcγR interactions were also crucial for the therapeutic activity of bnAbs in a post-exposure prophylaxis setting interfering with the establishment of a silent reservoir and reducing viremia in a therapeutic setting (Bournazos et al. 2014b; Halper-Stromberg et al. 2014). Engagement of activating type I FcγRs by bnAbs has further shown to result in the accelerated clearance of HIV-infected CD4$^+$ T cells (Lu et al. 2016). The engagement of FcγRs by bnAbs thus enables the immune system to combat HIV infection at various stages of the viral life cycle. A comprehensive analysis of the RV144 Thai Trial, the only trial demonstrating modest vaccine efficacy to date, revealed an important role for non-neutralizing antibodies and FcγR-mediated effector functions as a correlate of protection, further highlighting the important role of FcγRs for antibody-mediated protection irrespective of neutralization capacity (Pollara et al. 2017).

4.1.3 Respiratory Syncytial Virus

Palivizumab, a humanized IgG1 mAb recognizing a conserved neutralizing epitope of the F glycoprotein of respiratory syncytial virus (RSV), shows potent in vitro and in vivo activity and is now used for immunoprophylaxis in at-risk neonates (Johnson et al. 1997). A recent study demonstrated that efficient FcγR engagement by palivizumab is crucial for its protective capacity in vivo (Hiatt et al. 2014). Compared to the parental antibody, afucosylated palivizumab with enhanced affinity for FcγRIII resulted in about threefold lower RSV lung titers in a cotton rat challenge model, whereas an IgG2 variant of palivizumab, unable to efficiently engage FcγRs, only showed minimal viral control in vivo.

4.1.4 West Nile Virus

Murine mAbs directed against the nonstructural-1 (NS-1) protein of West Nile virus (WNV), a nonstructural secreted glycoprotein absent on virions but associated with the plasma membrane of infected cells, have been shown to mediate FcγR-dependent clearance of WNV-infected cells and protection from lethal WNV infection (Chung et al. 2006, 2007). Protection by NS1-specific mAbs required the engagement of activating FcγRs but not the presence of NK cells suggesting that ADCP is the main FcγR-mediated effector function in this model (Chung et al. 2007). Furthermore, a mAb directed against the NS-1 protein of Yellow Fever virus also required efficient FcγR engagement to protect mice against viral encephalitis (Schlesinger et al. 1993).

4.2 Bacteria

4.2.1 Bacillus Anthracis

Anthrax toxin neutralization assays using macrophage-like FcγR-expressing cell lines such as J774A.1 and RAW264.7 represent a unique in vitro setting to address the role of FcγR-dependent neutralization in vitro and demonstrate the important role of FcγRs for neutralization of *Bacillus anthracis* lethal toxin by polyclonal and monoclonal antibody preparations (Abboud et al. 2010; Verma et al. 2009). The in vitro and in vivo neutralizing capacity of a mAb directed against the protective antigen component of the lethal toxin (19D9) critically depended on the engagement of activating type I FcγRs with mAb isotype variants exhibiting higher affinity for activating FcγRs being more potent neutralizers (Abboud et al. 2010; Verma et al. 2009). A subsequent study generated a humanized version of 19D9 selectively engaging activating human FcγRs and performed *B. anthracis* challenge studies in a mouse model recapitulating human FcγR expression, which further demonstrated the importance of optimal engagement of activating FcγRs for antibody-mediated toxin neutralization (Bournazos et al. 2014a).

4.2.2 Bordetella Pertussis

The engagement of activating FcRs by antibodies specific for *Bordetella pertussis*, the causative agent of pertussis, can contribute to the clearance of bacteria from the respiratory tract of infected mice (Hellwig et al. 2001a, b). The engagement of activating FcγRs such as FcγRIII is important for bacterial clearance as mice challenged with *B. pertussis* opsonized with a bispecific mAb targeting FcγRII/III showed improved bacterial control, whereas a mAb targeting the complement receptor CD11b provided no benefit (Hellwig et al. 2001a). Furthermore, the results obtained in a human FcαRI-transgenic mouse model using immune serum IgA or a bispecific Ab targeting hFcαRI suggest that engagement of FcαRI can also contribute to bacterial clearance (Hellwig et al. 2001b). FcR-mediated phagocytosis of both IgG- and IgA-opsonized *B. pertussis* triggered an efficient oxidative burst in human polymorphonuclear leukocytes and simultaneous engagement of FcγRs and FcαR has been shown to result in enhanced phagocytosis (Rodriguez et al. 2001).

4.2.3 *Chlamydia Trachomatis*

FcγR-mediated effector mechanisms can contribute to the clearance of secondary infections with the intracellular bacterium *Chlamydia muridarum*, the murine genital infection model recapitulating many aspects of *Chlamydia trachomatis* infection in humans (Moore et al. 2002). Subsequent studies showed that mice lacking FcγRs mounted reduced Th1 responses upon reinfection due to limited antigen presentation by FcγR-deficient APCs and that CD4-derived IFNγ was crucial for efficient antibody-mediated pathogen clearance by neutrophils (Moore et al. 2003; Naglak et al. 2016, 2017).

4.2.4 *Legionella Pneumophila*

Antibodies directed against *Legionella pneumophila*, the causative agent of Legionnaires' disease, have shown to protect mice by promoting the lysosomal fusion of phagosomes containing opsonized bacteria in a FcγR-dependent manner (Joller et al. 2010). Phagocytic uptake of *L. pneumophila* by macrophages in the absence of FcγR signaling allows the pathogen to arrest phagolysosomal maturation by secretion of bacterial effector proteins into the cytoplasm thus establishing a replication-permissive vacuole. Signaling through activating FcγRs, however, renders host cells resistant and efficiently targets pathogens for lysosomal degradation. Experiments using isotype variants of *L. pneumophila*-specific mAb further demonstrated that isotypes efficiently engaging activating FcγRs (e.g., mouse IgG2c) provided improved protection compared with an isotype poorly engaging activating FcγRs (mouse IgG3) (Weber et al. 2014). Enhanced lysosomal targeting of opsonized pathogens might also contribute to the protection against other intracellular bacteria, which have evolved strategies to prevent phagolysosomal maturation and establish replication-permissive vacuoles.

4.2.5 *Mycobacterium Tuberculosis*

FcRs have also been implicated in regulating the immune response to *Mycobacterium tuberculosis* and ultimately bacterial burden. Mice lacking the inhibitory FcγRIIb showed elevated Th1 responses and reduced bacterial burden in the lungs, whereas mice lacking activating FcγRs demonstrated increased bacterial burden and succumbed faster to infection (Maglione et al. 2008). Furthermore, data obtained in a human FcαRI-transgenic mouse model also suggest that engagement of FcαRI by a *M. tuberculosis*-specific monoclonal IgA delivered intranasally in combination with IFNγ can reduce bacterial burden (Balu et al. 2011).

4.2.6 *Rickettsia Conorii*

Passive transfer of polyclonal immune serum and outer membrane protein A/B-specific mAbs but not Fab fragments protected immunodeficient mice from fatal infection with the intracellular gram-negative bacterium *Rickettsia conorii*, the causative agent of Boutonneuse fever, suggesting the involvement of FcγRs in antibody-mediated protection (Feng et al. 2004a). Opsonization of *R. conorii* with IgG diminished bacterial escape from phagosomes and triggered the generation of reactive oxygen and nitrogen species mediating killing of internalized pathogens (Feng et al. 2004b). Although this study did not utilize genetic models to address the specific role of FcγRs in this process, FcγRs are likely preventing phagosomal escape and mediate intracellular killing of opsonized *R. conorii* in a comparable manner as described for *Francisella tularensis*, an intracellular gram-negative bacterium and the causative agent of tularemia (Geier and Celli 2011).

4.2.7 *Salmonella Enterica*

The intracellular gram-negative bacterium *Salmonella enterica* serovar Typhimurium (ST), the causative agent of typhoid disease in mouse models, has evolved strategies allowing it to survive within phagocytic cells such as macrophages and DCs and establish replication-permissive vacuoles by preventing fusion with lysosomes. However, the engagement of the activating FcγRIII on DCs by IgG-opsonized ST has been shown to prevent bacterial escape by mediating efficient lysosomal targeting and subsequent degradation of bacteria (Tobar et al. 2004; Herrada et al. 2007). Furthermore, FcγRIII-mediated uptake and lysosomal targeting of opsonized ST resulted in efficient antigen processing and presentation, and could efficiently activate CD4$^+$ and CD8$^+$ T cells in vitro, suggesting that FcγR engagement can contribute to the generation of an antibacterial T cell response. Interestingly, although mice deficient for FcγRI-III initially exhibited higher bacterial loads upon immunization with a live-attenuated ST strain, they could efficiently mount cellular and humoral responses toward ST but succumbed to a subsequent high-dose challenge with a virulent strain (Menager et al. 2007). Overall, these data show that FcγRs play a crucial role in the control of ST infection.

4.2.8 *Staphylococcus Aureus*

Staphylococcus aureus is a gram-positive bacterium that can cause life-threating infections, and methicillin-resistant *S. aureus* represents a major public health concern. Neutralizing mAbs against staphylococcal enterotoxin B (SEB), one of the most potent known superantigens, can protect mice against lethal sepsis following intravenous challenge with *S. aureus* and result in a modest reduction of bacterial burden in skin abscesses (Varshney et al. 2011, 2013). A subsequent study testing the protective capacity of isotype switch variants (IgG1, IgG2a, and IgG2b) of a neutralizing SEB-specific mAb showed comparable in vitro neutralization potency but enhanced in vivo protection by the IgG2a variant, especially at lower doses, suggesting that efficient engagement of activating FcγRs is required for optimal in vivo activity (Varshney et al. 2014).

In addition to binding IgG, human FcγRs can also interact with members of the pentraxin family such as human serum amyloid P (SAP) and C-reactive protein (CRP), which are soluble innate pattern recognition molecules that can bind to microbial pathogens (Lu et al. 2008). Furthermore, FcαRI has been shown to interact with SAP and CRP (Lu et al. 2011). The engagement of FcRs by SAP and CRP can trigger comparable downstream signaling events and cellular responses as engagement by IgG or IgA (Lu et al. 2008,2011). SAP can bind to peptidoglycan and promote the phagocytosis of tagO-deficient *S. aureus* in a FcγR-dependent manner (An et al. 2013). However, the in vivo role of pentraxin/FcR interactions for antimicrobial protection is not well characterized.

4.2.9 *Streptococcus pneumoniae*

FcγRs play an important role in antibody-mediated protection and regulation of the immune response to *Streptococcus pneumoniae*. The expression of the inhibitory FcγRIIb is important for a balanced immune response and prevented septic shock and death of immunized mice following high-dose *S. pneumoniae* challenge (Clatworthy and Smith 2004). However, in a primary low-dose infection setting, global FcγRIIb deficiency conferred a survival advantage, whereas macrophage-specific overexpression of FcγRIIb was shown to reduce survival under these conditions (Clatworthy and Smith 2004; Brownlie et al. 2008). Engagement of FcγRIIb is thus important to balance efficient pathogen clearance and the release of septic shock cytokines with the ultimate goal of maximizing survival.

Engagement of FcγRs is crucial for the in vivo protective capacity of mAbs against the pneumococcal capsular polysaccharide (PPS) of *S. pneumoniae* (Tian et al. 2009). Interestingly, the ability of PPS-specific mouse IgG1 mAbs to promote *S. pneumoniae* killing in an in vitro opsonophagocytic killing assay (OPKA) failed to predict the in vivo protective capacity as a nonopsonic antibody efficiently protected mice in a FcγR-dependent manner (Tian et al. 2009). Furthermore, the requirements for antibody-mediated protection in vivo differ significantly between these mAbs, as opsonic mAbs required the presence of neutrophils and FcγRIIb, whereas as a nonopsonic mAb required macrophages and FcγRIII (Tian et al. 2009; Weber et al. 2012). These data further show that, although certain in vitro assays such as OPKA rely on FcγR engagement, they fail to recapitulate all FcγR-mediated effector functions contributing to in vivo protection.

4.3 Fungi and Parasites

4.3.1 Leishmania

FcγRs have been shown to play a crucial role during the infection with protozoan intracellular *Leishmania* parasites. Whereas early during infection *Leishmania major* was predominantly phagocytosed in a complement-dependent manner by macrophages, once the infection was established and parasite-specific IgG production induced, DCs efficiently phagocytosed parasites in an activating FcγR-dependent manner (Woelbing et al. 2006). FcγR-mediated uptake of IgG-opsonized parasites by DCs resulted in the efficient priming of Th1 cells and CD8$^+$ T cells, whereas mice lacking antibodies or activating FcγRs failed to mount efficient T cell responses resulting in increased lesion progression and higher parasite burden (Woelbing et al. 2006). In contrast to the data obtained with mice on the resistant C57BL6 background demonstrating a beneficial role of FcγRs, susceptible BALB/c mice lacking activating FcγRs have been shown to exhibit increased parasite control suggesting that the genetic background determines the role of activating FcγRs in *L. major* pathogenesis (Padigel and Farrell 2005).

4.3.2 Toxoplasma Gondii

FcγR-mediated processes such as ADCP are likely involved in host resistance to infection with the intracellular protozoan parasite *Toxoplasma gondii*. FcγR-mediated phagocytosis of opsonized parasites has been shown to result in efficient lysosomal targeting preventing replication of the parasite within the cell (Joiner et al. 1990). A similar process was described and attributed to contribute to resistance against *Encephalitozoon cuniculi*, an intracellular fungus (Niederkorn and Shadduck 1980). Although the in vivo role of FcγRs for resistance against *T. gondii* has not been directly addressed so far, immune IgG transfer experiments in B cell deficient mice demonstrated that antibody-mediated effector functions also contribute to in vivo resistance (Kang et al. 2000).

4.3.3 Schistosoma Mansoni

IgE/FcεRI interactions may play a central role in resistance to infections with parasitic helminths such as *Schistosoma mansoni*, one of the causative agents of

Schistosomiasis. IgE can mediate killing of *S. mansoni* larvae by macrophages, eosinophils, and platelets in vitro (Joseph et al. 1983; Butterworth 1984). IgE-mediated killing of *Acanthocheilonema viteae*, a filarial parasitic nematode, by macrophages and eosinophils in vitro further supports the role of IgE as the central mediator for ADCC against parasitic worms (Haque et al. 1981). Human macrophages, eosinophils, and platelets express the high-affinity IgE FcεRI, which has been shown to be important for IgE-mediated killing in vitro (Gounni et al. 1994). However, species-specific differences in the expression pattern of FcεRI have hampered studies addressing the in vivo role of the IgE/FcεRI interaction in murine *S. mansoni* infection models and might thus explain conflicting results. Whereas mice deficient for IgE were more susceptible for infection with *S. mansoni* and had higher worm burden, FcεRI deficiency did not affect worm burden (King et al. 1997; Jankovic et al. 1997). The use of hFcεRI-transgenic mouse models reflecting the human expression pattern of hFcεRI might help to elucidate the in vivo role of IgE/FcεRI interactions during *S. mansoni* infection.

4.3.4 *Cryptococcus Neoformans*

The efficient engagement of activating FcγRs by mAbs directed against the capsular polyssacharide (cPS) has been shown to contribute to protection against *Cryptococcus neoformans*, a fungus infecting mainly immunocompromised patients and causing meningitis. The opsonic activity of cPS-specific mAbs in vitro crucially depends on the isotype of the antibody, with mouse IgG2a being the most potent isotype (Schlageter and Kozel 1990). Furthermore, therapeutic application of IgG2a and IgG2b variants of a cPS-specific mAb to mice challenged with a highly pathogenic strain of *C. neoformans* resulted in reduced yeast burden in spleen and lungs; however, it failed to ultimately reduce yeast burden in brain and prevent death (Sanford et al. 1990). Engagement of activating FcγRs has been shown to be important for the in vivo protective capacity of a cPS-specific IgG1 mAb and resulted in enhanced survival, whereas an IgG3 variant with identical specificity enhanced pathogenicity in vivo independent of activating FcγRs (Yuan et al. 1998). These data demonstrate that the isotype and efficient engagement of FcγRs in vivo are crucial for the protective capacity of *C. neoformans*-specific antibodies.

5 Microbial Evasion Strategies

Although Fc–FcγR interactions can mediate effective antimicrobial protection in vivo, a wide range of pathogens has developed sophisticated evasion mechanisms. Pathogenic bacteria have evolved several evasion mechanisms including Fc-binding proteins such as protein A/G (Foster 2005), IgG-cleaving enzymes such as IdeS (Von Pawel-Rammingen et al. 2002), IgG-specific endoglycosidases such as EndoS (Collin and Olsen 2001), and injection of phagocytosis inhibitors into phagocytic cells (Marches et al. 2008). Various viruses can also interfere with FcγR-mediated effector mechanisms through expression of viral FcγRs and viral homologs of immunoregulatory proteins on the surface of infected cells (Lubinski et al. 2011; Cameron et al. 2005).

In addition to direct microbial evasion strategies requiring the expression of specific evasion proteins, pathogens may also exploit dysfunctions of the immune system that occur during persistent infections, autoimmune diseases, and cancer. We and others have recently shown that excessive immune complex formation in mice persistently infected with lymphocytic choriomeningitis virus (LCMV) interferes with various FcγR-mediated antibody effector functions without negatively affecting the overall expression pattern of FcγRs on effector cells (Fig. 3) (Wieland et al. 2015; Yamada et al. 2015). The inhibition of FcγR-mediated antibody effector functions is due to immune complex formation and not the persistent viral infection per se, as persistently infected mice in the absence of an antiviral B cell response or with a strikingly diminished antiviral B cell response exhibit normal FcγR-mediated effector functions. During persistent LCMV infection, immune complexes inhibit several FcγR-mediated effector functions such as ADCC of infected cells, ADCP of antibody-coated target cells, antigen cross-presentation to $CD8^+$ T cells, and also abrogate the therapeutic activity of depleting and agonistic antibodies relying on the efficient engagement of FcγRs (Wieland et al. 2015; Yamada et al. 2015).

Elevated levels of circulating immune complexes as well as deposition in the kidney have been reported in various diseases ranging from persistent viral infections such as B virus, hepatitis C virus and HIV, to autoimmune diseases and cancer (Johnson et al. 1993; Tsai et al. 1995; Nobakht et al. 2016; Lefaucheur et al. 2006; Theofilopoulos et al. 1977). Excessive immune complex formation has been shown to inhibit the therapeutic activity of rituximab, a chimeric anti-human CD20 widely used for B cell malignancies and autoimmune diseases, during persistent LCMV infection as well as in a murine lupus model (Wieland et al. 2015; Yamada et al. 2015; Ahuja et al. 2011). The proposed mechanism of reduced FcγR engagement due to excessive immune complex formation might thus explain the observed variation in B cell depletion efficacy in systemic lupus erythematosus patients upon rituximab treatment (Looney et al. 2004). Overall, these studies show that circulating immune complexes occur in various diseases and can result in significant interference with FcγR-mediated antibody effector functions, potentially favoring infections despite the presence of humoral immunity and contributing to viral persistence.

We have recently shown that endogenous immune complexes do not simply abrogate the engagement of FcγRs by depleting antibodies but rather compete with depleting antibodies for binding to FcγRs, increasing the apparent threshold required for the efficient induction of FcγR-mediated effector functions (Wieland et al. 2018). Efficient antibody-mediated depletion in the presence of competing endogenous immune complexes can be achieved by targeting highly expressed surface antigens such as CD90 or by using antibodies with Fc domain modifications such as afucosylation that are aimed at increasing the affinity to activating FcγRs (Fig. 3). Overall, our data demonstrate that excessive immune complex formation

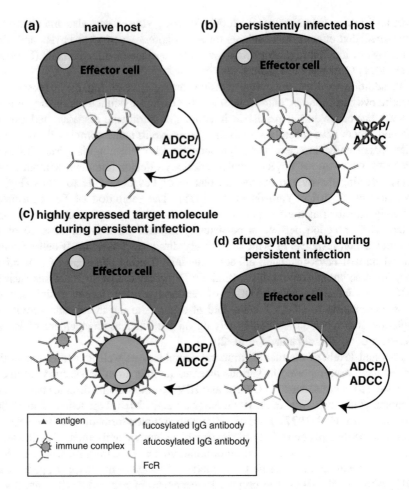

Fig. 3 Differential requirements for the efficient induction of antibody-dependent cellular phagocytosis (ADCP) and antibody-dependent cellular cytotoxicity (ADCC) in naïve and persistently infected hosts. **a** Efficient ADCP/ADCC in naïve hosts. **b** Immune complexes prevent efficient ADCP/ADCC in persistently infected hosts. **c** Highly opsonized targets can outcompete endogenous immune complexes efficiently triggering ADCP/ADCC. **d** Afucosylated mAbs with increased affinity for activating FcγRs can outcompete endogenous immune complexes and efficiently trigger ADCP/ADCC during persistent infection

can be an obstacle for therapeutic antibodies to efficiently engage FcγRs but can be overcome by selectively targeting highly abundant surface antigens or the use of Fc-engineered monoclonal antibodies. Future experiments using co-infection models will reveal the effects of excessive immune complex formation on antibody-mediated antimicrobial protection in vivo. Furthermore, these experiments will allow optimization of antibody-based antimicrobial intervention strategies.

6 Conclusions

FcRs mediate direct antimicrobial protection by various effector mechanisms and are involved in the regulation of a plethora of immunological processes which indirectly contribute to antimicrobial protection. Using knockout mouse models as well as Fc-engineered antibodies, studies in various infection models demonstrate that many pathogen-specific antibodies rely on efficient FcγR engagement for optimal antimicrobial protection in vivo. Most notably, the initially surprising observations that broadly neutralizing antibodies against various pathogens such as Influenza virus and HIV need to engage activating FcγRs for optimal in vivo protection have important implications for the development of therapeutics and vaccines. The induction of protective broadly neutralizing antibody responses may thus require the induction of antibodies of a particular specificity and IgG isotype.

While some in vitro assays rely on Fc–FcγR interactions to assess protective antibody responses, these assays fail to recapitulate the complex landscape of cellular FcγR expression. Thus, in vivo experiments are ultimately required to assess the role of Fc–FcγR interactions for antimicrobial protection. Future studies assessing the protective capacity of human mAbs in vivo should thus be performed in human FcγR transgenic mice that accurately reflect the cellular FcγR expression pattern in humans.

References

Abboud N, Chow SK, Saylor C, Janda A, Ravetch JV, Scharff MD, Casadevall A (2010) A requirement for FcγR in antibody-mediated bacterial toxin neutralization. J Exp Med 207:2395–2405

Abu-Ghazaleh RI, Fujisawa T, Mestecky J, Kyle RA, Gleich GJ (1989) IgA-induced eosinophil degranulation. J Immunol 142:2393–2400

Ahuja A, Teichmann LL, Wang H, Dunn R, Kehry MR, Shlomchik MJ (2011) An acquired defect in IgG-dependent phagocytosis explains the impairment in antibody-mediated cellular depletion in Lupus. J Immunol 187:3888–3894

Amigorena S, Bonnerot C, Drake JR, Choquet D, Hunziker W, Guillet JG, Webster P, Sautes C, Mellman I, Fridman WH (1992a) Cytoplasmic domain heterogeneity and functions of IgG Fc receptors in B lymphocytes. Science 256:1808–1812

Amigorena S, Salamero J, Davoust J, Fridman WH, Bonnerot C (1992b) Tyrosine-containing motif that transduces cell activation signals also determines internalization and antigen presentation via type III receptors for IgG. Nature 358:337–341

An JH, Kurokawa K, Jung DJ, Kim MJ, Kim CH, Fujimoto Y, Fukase K, Coggeshall KM, Lee BL (2013) Human SAP is a novel peptidoglycan recognition protein that induces complement-independent phagocytosis of *Staphylococcus aureus*. J Immunol 191:3319–3327

Anthony RM, Kobayashi T, Wermeling F, Ravetch JV (2011) Intravenous γglobulin suppresses inflammation through a novel T(H)2 pathway. Nature 475:110–113

Araki N, Johnson MT, Swanson JA (1996) A role for phosphoinositide 3-kinase in the completion of macropinocytosis and phagocytosis by macrophages. J Cell Biol 135:1249–1260

Balu S, Reljic R, Lewis MJ, Pleass RJ, McIntosh R, van Kooten C, van Egmond M, Challacombe S, Woof JM, Ivanyi J (2011) A novel human IgA monoclonal antibody protects against tuberculosis. J Immunol 186:3113–3119

Bergtold A, Desai DD, Gavhane A, Clynes R (2005) Cell surface recycling of internalized antigen permits dendritic cell priming of B cells. Immunity 23:503–514

Bidgood SR, Tam JC, McEwan WA, Mallery DL, James LC (2014) Translocated IgA mediates neutralization and stimulates innate immunity inside infected cells. Proc Natl Acad Sci U S A 111:13463–13468

Bolland S, Ravetch JV (2000) Spontaneous autoimmune disease in Fc(γ)RIIB-deficient mice results from strain-specific epistasis. Immunity 13:277–285

Bolland S, Yim YS, Tus K, Wakeland EK, Ravetch JV (2002) Genetic modifiers of systemic lupus erythematosus in FcγRIIB(−/−) mice. J Exp Med 195:1167–1174

Boruchov AM, Heller G, Veri MC, Bonvini E, Ravetch JV, Young JW (2005) Activating and inhibitory IgG Fc receptors on human DCs mediate opposing functions. J Clin Invest 115:2914–2923

Bournazos S, Chow SK, Abboud N, Casadevall A, Ravetch JV (2014a) Human IgG Fc domain engineering enhances antitoxin neutralizing antibody activity. J Clin Invest 124:725–729

Bournazos S, Klein F, Pietzsch J, Seaman MS, Nussenzweig MC, Ravetch JV (2014b) Broadly neutralizing anti-HIV-1 antibodies require Fc effector functions for in vivo activity. Cell 158:1243–1253

Bournazos S, Ravetch JV (2015) Fcγ receptor pathways during active and passive immunization. Immunol Rev 268:88–103

Bournazos S, Wang TT, Dahan R, Maamary J, Ravetch JV (2017) Signaling by antibodies: recent progress. Annu Rev Immunol 35:285–311

Bournazos S, Wang TT, Ravetch JV (2016) The role and function of fcγ receptors on myeloid cells. Microbiol Spectr, 4

Brownlie RJ, Lawlor KE, Niederer HA, Cutler AJ, Xiang Z, Clatworthy MR, Floto RA, Greaves DR, Lyons PA, Smith KG (2008) Distinct cell-specific control of autoimmunity and infection by FcγRIIb. J Exp Med 205:883–895

Butterworth AE (1984) Cell-mediated damage to helminths. Adv Parasitol 23:143–235

Cameron CM, Barrett JW, Mann M, Lucas A, McFadden G (2005) Myxoma virus M128L is expressed as a cell surface CD47-like virulence factor that contributes to the downregulation of macrophage activation in vivo. Virology 337:55–67

Caron E, Hall A (1998) Identification of two distinct mechanisms of phagocytosis controlled by different Rho GTPases. Science 282:1717–1721

Chung KM, Nybakken GE, Thompson BS, Engle MJ, Marri A, Fremont DH, Diamond MS (2006) Antibodies against West Nile Virus nonstructural protein NS1 prevent lethal infection through Fc γ receptor-dependent and -independent mechanisms. J Virol 80:1340–1351

Chung KM, Thompson BS, Fremont DH, Diamond MS (2007) Antibody recognition of cell surface-associated NS1 triggers Fc-γ receptor-mediated phagocytosis and clearance of West Nile Virus-infected cells. J Virol 81:9551–9555

Clatworthy MR, Smith KG (2004) FcγRIIb balances efficient pathogen clearance and the cytokine-mediated consequences of sepsis. J Exp Med 199:717–723

Clynes R, Maizes JS, Guinamard R, Ono M, Takai T, Ravetch JV (1999) Modulation of immune complex-induced inflammation in vivo by the coordinate expression of activation and inhibitory Fc receptors. J Exp Med 189:179–185

Collin M, Olsen A (2001) EndoS, a novel secreted protein from Streptococcus pyogenes with endoglycosidase activity on human IgG. EMBO J 20:3046–3055

Corti D, Voss J, Gamblin SJ, Codoni G, Macagno A, Jarrossay D, Vachieri SG, Pinna D, Minola A, Vanzetta F, Silacci C, Fernandez-Rodriguez BM, Agatic G, Bianchi S, Giacchetto-Sasselli I, Calder L, Sallusto F, Collins P, Haire LF, Temperton N, Langedijk JP, Skehel JJ, Lanzavecchia A (2011) A neutralizing antibody selected from plasma cells that binds to group 1 and group 2 influenza A hemagglutinins. Science 333:850–856

Cox D, Tseng CC, Bjekic G, Greenberg S (1999) A requirement for phosphatidylinositol 3-kinase in pseudopod extension. J Biol Chem 274:1240–1247

Crowley MT, Costello PS, Fitzer-Attas CJ, Turner M, Meng F, Lowell C, Tybulewicz VL, Defranco AL (1997) A critical role for Syk in signal transduction and phagocytosis mediated by Fcγ receptors on macrophages. J Exp Med 186:1027–1039

de Saint Basile G, Ménasché G, Fischer A (2010) Molecular mechanisms of biogenesis and exocytosis of cytotoxic granules. Nat Rev Immunol 10(8):568

Desjardins M, Huber LA, Parton RG, Griffiths G (1994) Biogenesis of phagolysosomes proceeds through a sequential series of interactions with the endocytic apparatus. J Cell Biol 124:677–688

Dhodapkar KM, Krasovsky J, Williamson B, Dhodapkar MV (2002) Antitumor monoclonal antibodies enhance cross-presentation of Cellular antigens and the generation of myeloma-specific killer T cells by dendritic cells. J Exp Med 195:125–133

Dilillo DJ, Palese P, Wilson PC, Ravetch JV (2016) Broadly neutralizing anti-influenza antibodies require Fc receptor engagement for in vivo protection. J Clin Invest 126:605–610

Dilillo DJ, Tan GS, Palese P, Ravetch JV (2014) Broadly neutralizing hemagglutinin stalk-specific antibodies require FcγR interactions for protection against influenza virus in vivo. Nat Med 20:143–151

Dombrowicz D, Quatannens B, Papin JP, Capron A, Capron M (2000) Expression of a functional Fc epsilon RI on rat eosinophils and macrophages. J Immunol 165:1266–1271

Dugast AS, Tonelli A, Berger CT, Ackerman ME, Sciaranghella G, Liu Q, Sips M, Toth I, Piechocka-Trocha A, Ghebremichael M, Alter G (2011) Decreased Fc receptor expression on innate immune cells is associated with impaired antibody-mediated cellular phagocytic activity in chronically HIV-1 infected individuals. Virology 415:160–167

Durden DL, Kim HM, Calore B, Liu Y (1995) The Fc γ RI receptor signals through the activation of hck and MAP kinase. J Immunol 154:4039–4047

Eischen CM, Schilling JD, Lynch DH, Krammer PH, Leibson PJ (1996) Fc receptor-induced expression of Fas ligand on activated NK cells facilitates cell-mediated cytotoxicity and subsequent autocrine NK cell apoptosis. J Immunol 156:2693–2699

Ekiert DC, Bhabha G, Elsliger MA, Friesen RH, Jongeneelen M, Throsby M, Goudsmit J, Wilson IA (2009) Antibody recognition of a highly conserved influenza virus epitope. Science 324:246–251

el Bakkouri K, Descamps F, de Filette M, Smet A, Festjens E, Birkett A, van Rooijen N, Verbeek S, Fiers W, Saelens X (2011) Universal vaccine based on ectodomain of matrix protein 2 of influenza A: Fc receptors and alveolar macrophages mediate protection. J Immunol 186:1022–1031

Fabian I, Kletter Y, Mor S, Geller-Bernstein C, Ben-Yaakov M, Volovitz B, Golde DW (1992) Activation of human eosinophil and neutrophil functions by haematopoietic growth factors: comparisons of IL-1, IL-3, IL-5 and GM-CSF. Br J Haematol 80:137–143

Feng HM, Whitworth T, Olano JP, Popov VL, Walker DH (2004a) Fc-dependent polyclonal antibodies and antibodies to outer membrane proteins A and B, but not to lipopolysaccharide, protect SCID mice against fatal *Rickettsia conorii* infection. Infect Immun 72:2222–2228

Feng HM, Whitworth T, Popov V, Walker DH (2004b) Effect of antibody on the rickettsia-host cell interaction. Infect Immun 72:3524–3530

Fiebiger BM, Maamary J, Pincetic A, Ravetch JV (2015) Protection in antibody- and T cell-mediated autoimmune diseases by antiinflammatory IgG Fcs requires type II FcRs. Proc Natl Acad Sci U S A 112:E2385–E2394

Flannagan RS, Jaumouille V, Grinstein S (2012) The cell biology of phagocytosis. Annu Rev Pathol 7:61–98

Forthal DN, Landucci G, Bream J, Jacobson LP, Phan TB, Montoya B (2007) FcγRIIa genotype predicts progression of HIV infection. J Immunol 179:7916–7923

Foster TJ (2005) Immune evasion by staphylococci. Nat Rev Microbiol 3:948–958

Fu SL, Pierre J, Smith-Norowitz TA, Hagler M, Bowne W, Pincus MR, Mueller CM, Zenilman ME, Bluth MH (2008) Immunoglobulin E antibodies from pancreatic cancer patients mediate antibody-dependent cell-mediated cytotoxicity against pancreatic cancer cells. Clin Exp Immunol 153:401–409

Ganesan LP, Fang H, Marsh CB, Tridandapani S (2003) The protein-tyrosine phosphatase SHP-1 associates with the phosphorylated immunoreceptor tyrosine-based activation motif of Fc γ RIIa to modulate signaling events in myeloid cells. J Biol Chem 278:35710–35717

Geier H, Celli J (2011) Phagocytic receptors dictate phagosomal escape and intracellular proliferation of *Francisella tularensis*. Infect Immun 79:2204–2214

Gounni AS, Lamkhioued B, Ochiai K, Tanaka Y, Delaporte E, Capron A, Kinet JP, Capron M (1994) High-affinity IgE receptor on eosinophils is involved in defence against parasites. Nature 367:183–186

Griffin FM, Griffin JA, Leider JE, Silverstein SC (1975) Studies on the mechanism of phagocytosis. I. Requirements for circumferential attachment of particle-bound ligands to specific receptors on the macrophage plasma membrane. J Exp Med 142(5):1263–1282

Guilliams M, Bruhns P, Saeys Y, Hammad H, Lambrecht BN (2014) The function of Fcγ receptors in dendritic cells and macrophages. Nat Rev Immunol 14:94–108

Halper-Stromberg A, Lu CL, Klein F, Horwitz JA, Bournazos S, Nogueira L, Eisenreich TR, Liu C, Gazumyan A, Schaefer U, Furze RC, Seaman MS, Prinjha R, Tarakhovsky A, Ravetch JV, Nussenzweig MC (2014) Broadly neutralizing antibodies and viral inducers decrease rebound from HIV-1 latent reservoirs in humanized mice. Cell 158:989–999

Hamada F, Aoki M, Akiyama T, Toyoshima K (1993) Association of immunoglobulin G Fc receptor II with Src-like protein-tyrosine kinase Fgr in neutrophils. Proc Natl Acad Sci U S A 90:6305–6309

Hamawy MM, Minoguchi K, Swaim WD, Mergenhagen SE, Siraganian RP (1995) A 77-kDa protein associates with pp125FAK in mast cells and becomes tyrosine-phosphorylated by high affinity IgE receptor aggregation. J Biol Chem 270:12305–12309

Haque A, Ouaissi A, Joseph M, Capron M, Capron A (1981) IgE antibody in eosinophil- and macrophage-mediated in vitro killing of Dipetalonema viteae microfilariae. J Immunol 127:716–725

Hauler F, Mallery DL, McEwan WA, Bidgood SR, James LC (2012) AAA ATPase p97/VCP is essential for TRIM21-mediated virus neutralization. Proc Natl Acad Sci U S A 109:19733–19738

Hellwig SM, van Oirschot HF, Hazenbos WL, van Spriel AB, Mooi FR, van de Winkel JG (2001a) Targeting to Fcγ receptors, but not CR3 (CD11b/CD18), increases clearance of Bordetella pertussis. J Infect Dis 183:871–879

Hellwig SM, van Spriel AB, Schellekens JF, Mooi FR, van de Winkel JG (2001b) Immunoglobulin A-mediated protection against Bordetella pertussis infection. Infect Immun 69:4846–4850

Herrada AA, Contreras FJ, Tobar JA, Pacheco R, Kalergis AM (2007) Immune complex-induced enhancement of bacterial antigen presentation requires Fcγ receptor III expression on dendritic cells. Proc Natl Acad Sci U S A 104:13402–13407

Hessell AJ, Hangartner L, Hunter M, Havenith CE, Beurskens FJ, Bakker JM, Lanigan CM, Landucci G, Forthal DN, Parren PW, Marx PA, Burton DR (2007) Fc receptor but not complement binding is important in antibody protection against HIV. Nature 449:101–104

Hiatt A, Bohorova N, Bohorov O, Goodman C, Kim D, Pauly MH, Velasco J, Whaley KJ, Piedra PA, Gilbert BE, Zeitlin L (2014) Glycan variants of a respiratory syncytial virus antibody with enhanced effector function and in vivo efficacy. Proc Natl Acad Sci U S A 111:5992–5997

Hoppe AD, Swanson JA (2004) Cdc42, Rac1, and Rac2 display distinct patterns of activation during phagocytosis. Mol Biol Cell 15:3509–3519

James LC, Keeble AH, Khan Z, Rhodes DA, Trowsdale J (2007) Structural basis for PRYSPRY-mediated tripartite motif (TRIM) protein function. Proc Natl Acad Sci U S A 104:6200–6205

Jankovic D, Kullberg MC, Dombrowicz D, Barbieri S, Caspar P, Wynn TA, Paul WE, Cheever AW, Kinet JP, Sher A (1997) Fc epsilonRI-deficient mice infected with *Schistosoma mansoni* mount normal Th2-type responses while displaying enhanced liver pathology. J Immunol 159:1868–1875

Johnson RJ, Gretch DR, Yamabe H, Hart J, Bacchi CE, Hartwell P, Couser WG, Corey L, Wener MH, Alpers CE et al (1993) Membranoproliferative glomerulonephritis associated with hepatitis C virus infection. New Engl J Med 328(7):465–470

Johnson S, Oliver C, Prince GA, Hemming VG, Pfarr DS, Wang SC, Dormitzer M, O'Grady J, Koenig S, Tamura JK, Woods R, Bansal G, Couchenour D, Tsao E, Hall WC, Young JF (1997) Development of a humanized monoclonal antibody (MEDI-493) with potent in vitro and in vivo activity against respiratory syncytial virus. J Infect Dis 176:1215–1224

Joiner KA, Fuhrman SA, Miettinen HM, Kasper LH, Mellman I (1990) *Toxoplasma gondii*: fusion competence of parasitophorous vacuoles in Fc receptor-transfected fibroblasts. Science 249:641–646

Joller N, Weber SS, Muller AJ, Sporri R, Selchow P, Sander P, Hilbi H, Oxenius A (2010) Antibodies protect against intracellular bacteria by Fc receptor-mediated lysosomal targeting. Proc Natl Acad Sci U S A 107:20441–20446

Jonsson F, Mancardi DA, Albanesi M, Bruhns P (2013) Neutrophils in local and systemic antibody-dependent inflammatory and anaphylactic reactions. J Leukoc Biol 94:643–656

Joseph M, Auriault C, Capron A, Vorng H, Viens P (1983) A new function for platelets: IgE-dependent killing of schistosomes. Nature 303:810–812

Jouvin MH, Adamczewski M, Numerof R, Letourneur O, Valle A, Kinet JP (1994) Differential control of the tyrosine kinases Lyn and Syk by the two signaling chains of the high affinity immunoglobulin E receptor. J Biol Chem 269:5918–5925

Kanakaraj P, Duckworth B, Azzoni L, Kamoun M, Cantley LC, Perussia B (1994) Phosphatidylinositol-3 kinase activation induced upon Fc γ RIIIA-ligand interaction. J Exp Med 179:551–558

Kang H, Remington JS, Suzuki Y (2000) Decreased resistance of B cell-deficient mice to infection with Toxoplasma gondii despite unimpaired expression of IFN-γ, TNF-alpha, and inducible nitric oxide synthase. J Immunol 164:2629–2634

Kant AM, De P, Peng X, Yi T, Rawlings DJ, Kim JS, Durden DL (2002) SHP-1 regulates Fcγ receptor-mediated phagocytosis and the activation of RAC. Blood 100:1852–1859

Kato T, Kitagawa S (2006) Regulation of neutrophil functions by proinflammatory cytokines. Int J Hematol 84:205–209

Keeble AH, Khan Z, Forster A, James LC (2008) TRIM21 is an IgG receptor that is structurally, thermodynamically, and kinetically conserved. Proc Natl Acad Sci U S A 105:6045–6050

Kiefer F, Brumell J, Al-Alawi N, Latour S, Cheng A, Veillette A, Grinstein S, Pawson T (1998) The Syk protein tyrosine kinase is essential for Fcγ receptor signaling in macrophages and neutrophils. Mol Cell Biol 18:4209–4220

King CL, Xianli J, Malhotra I, Liu S, Mahmoud AA, Oettgen HC (1997) Mice with a targeted deletion of the IgE gene have increased worm burdens and reduced granulomatous inflammation following primary infection with *Schistosoma mansoni*. J Immunol 158:294–300

Larsen EC, Ueyama T, Brannock PM, Shirai Y, Saito N, Larsson C, Loegering D, Weber PB, Lennartz MR (2002) A role for PKC-epsilon in Fc γR-mediated phagocytosis by RAW 264.7 cells. J Cell Biol 159:939–944

Lefaucheur, C., Stengel, B., Nochy, D., Martel, P., Hill, G. S., Jacquot, C., Rossert, J. & Group, G.-P. S (2006) Membranous nephropathy and cancer: epidemiologic evidence and determinants of high-risk cancer association. Kidney Int 70:1510–1517

Leon PE, He W, Mullarkey CE, Bailey MJ, Miller MS, Krammer F, Palese P, Tan GS (2016) Optimal activation of Fc-mediated effector functions by influenza virus hemagglutinin antibodies requires two points of contact. Proc Natl Acad Sci U S A 113:E5944–E5951

Liao F, Shin HS, Rhee SG (1992) Tyrosine phosphorylation of phospholipase C-γ 1 induced by cross-linking of the high-affinity or low-affinity Fc receptor for IgG in U937 cells. Proc Natl Acad Sci U S A 89:3659–3663

Looney RJ, Anolik JH, Campbell D, Felgar RE, Young F, Arend LJ, Sloand JA, Rosenblatt J, Sanz I (2004) B cell depletion as a novel treatment for systemic lupus erythematosus: a phase I/II dose-escalation trial of rituximab. Arthritis Rheum 50:2580–2589

Lorenzi R, Brickell PM, Katz DR, Kinnon C, Thrasher AJ (2000) Wiskott-Aldrich syndrome protein is necessary for efficient IgG-mediated phagocytosis. Blood 95:2943–2946

Lu CC, Wu TS, Hsu YJ, Chang CJ, Lin CS, Chia JH, Wu TL, Huang TT, Martel J, Ojcius DM, Young JD, Lai HC (2014) NK cells kill mycobacteria directly by releasing perforin and granulysin. J Leukoc Biol 96:1119–1129

Lu CL, Murakowski DK, Bournazos S, Schoofs T, Sarkar D, Halper-Stromberg A, Horwitz JA, Nogueira L, Golijanin J, Gazumyan A, Ravetch JV, Caskey M, Chakraborty AK, Nussenzweig MC (2016) Enhanced clearance of HIV-1-infected cells by broadly neutralizing antibodies against HIV-1 in vivo. Science 352:1001–1004

Lu J, Marjon KD, Marnell LL, Wang R, Mold C, du Clos TW, Sun P (2011) Recognition and functional activation of the human IgA receptor (FcalphaRI) by C-reactive protein. Proc Natl Acad Sci U S A 108:4974–4979

Lu J, Marnell LL, Marjon KD, Mold C, du Clos TW, Sun PD (2008) Structural recognition and functional activation of FcγR by innate pentraxins. Nature 456:989–992

Lubinski JM, Lazear HM, Awasthi S, Wang F, Friedman HM (2011) The herpes simplex virus 1 IgG fc receptor blocks antibody-mediated complement activation and antibody-dependent cellular cytotoxicity in vivo. J Virol 85:3239–3249

Maglione PJ, Xu J, Casadevall A, Chan J (2008) Fc γ receptors regulate immune activation and susceptibility during *Mycobacterium tuberculosis* infection. J Immunol 180:3329–3338

Mallery DL, McEwan WA, Bidgood SR, Towers GJ, Johnson CM, James LC (2010) Antibodies mediate intracellular immunity through tripartite motif-containing 21 (TRIM21). Proc Natl Acad Sci U S A 107:19985–19990

Manz RA, Thiel A, Radbruch A (1997) Lifetime of plasma cells in the bone marrow. Nature 388:133–134

Marches O, Covarelli V, Dahan S, Cougoule C, Bhatta P, Frankel G, Caron E (2008) EspJ of enteropathogenic and enterohaemorrhagic *Escherichia coli* inhibits opsono-phagocytosis. Cell Microbiol 10:1104–1115

May RC, Caron E, Hall A, Machesky LM (2000) Involvement of the Arp2/3 complex in phagocytosis mediated by FcγR or CR3. Nat Cell Biol 2:246–248

Mazor Y, Yang C, Borrok MJ, Ayriss J, Aherne K, Wu H, Dall'Acqua WF (2016) Enhancement of immune effector functions by modulating IgG's intrinsic affinity for target antigen. PLoS ONE 11:e0157788

McEwan WA, Hauler F, Williams CR, Bidgood SR, Mallery DL, Crowther RA, James LC (2012) Regulation of virus neutralization and the persistent fraction by TRIM21. J Virol 86:8482–8491

McEwan WA, Tam JC, Watkinson RE, Bidgood SR, Mallery DL, James LC (2013) Intracellular antibody-bound pathogens stimulate immune signaling via the Fc receptor TRIM21. Nat Immunol 14:327–336

Memoli MJ, Shaw PA, Han A, Czajkowski L, Reed S, Athota R, Bristol T, Fargis S, Risos K, Powers JH, Davey RT, Taubenberger JK (2016) Evaluation of antihemagglutinin and antineuraminidase antibodies as correlates of protection in an influenza A/H1N1 virus healthy human challenge model. MBio 7(2):e00416–e00417

Menager N, Foster G, Ugrinovic S, Uppington H, Verbeek S, Mastroeni P (2007) Fcγ receptors are crucial for the expression of acquired resistance to virulent *Salmonella enterica* serovar Typhimurium in vivo but are not required for the induction of humoral or T-cell-mediated immunity. Immunology 120:424–432

Moller E (1967) Cytotoxicity by nonimmune allogeneic lymphoid cells. Specific suppression by antibody treatment of the lymphoid cells. J Exp Med 126:395–405

Moore T, Ananaba GA, Bolier J, Bowers S, Belay T, Eko FO, Igietseme JU (2002) Fc receptor regulation of protective immunity against *Chlamydia trachomatis*. Immunology 105:213–221

Moore T, Ekworomadu CO, Eko FO, Macmillan L, Ramey K, Ananaba GA, Patrickson JW, Nagappan PR, Lyn D, Black CM, Igietseme JU (2003) Fc receptor-mediated antibody regulation of T cell immunity against intracellular pathogens. J Infect Dis 188:617–624

Morton HC, van Egmond M, van de Winkel JG (1996) Structure and function of human IgA Fc receptors (Fc alpha R). Crit Rev Immunol 16:423–440

Muta T, Kurosaki T, Misulovin Z, Sanchez M, Nussenzweig MC, Ravetch JV (1994) A 13-amino-acid motif in the cytoplasmic domain of Fc γ RIIB modulates B-cell receptor signalling. Nature 368:70–73

Naglak EK, Morrison SG, Morrison RP (2016). IFNγ is required for optimal antibody-mediated immunity against genital chlamydia infection. Infec Immun IAI-00749

Naglak EK, Morrison SG, Morrison RP (2017) Neutrophils are central to antibody-mediated protection against Genital Chlamydia. Infect Immun 85

Nakamura K, Malykhin A, Coggeshall KM (2002) The Src homology 2 domain-containing inositol 5-phosphatase negatively regulates Fcγ receptor-mediated phagocytosis through immunoreceptor tyrosine-based activation motif-bearing phagocytic receptors. Blood 100:3374–3382

Nathan C, Cunningham-Bussel A (2013) Beyond oxidative stress: an immunologist's guide to reactive oxygen species. Nat Rev Immunol 13:349–361

Niederkorn JY, Shadduck JA (1980) Role of antibody and complement in the control of Encephalitozoon cuniculi infections by rabbit macrophages. Infect Immun 27:995–1002

Nimmerjahn F, Ravetch JV (2005) Divergent immunoglobulin g subclass activity through selective Fc receptor binding. Science 310:1510–1512

Ninomiya N, Hazeki K, Fukui Y, Seya T, Okada T, Hazeki O, Ui M (1994) Involvement of phosphatidylinositol 3-kinase in Fc γ receptor signaling. J Biol Chem 269:22732–22737

Nobakht E, Cohen SD, Rosenberg AZ, Kimmel PL (2016) HIV-associated immune complex kidney disease. Nat Rev Nephrol 12:291–300

Odin JA, Edberg JC, Painter CJ, Kimberly RP, Unkeless JC (1991) Regulation of phagocytosis and [Ca2+]i flux by distinct regions of an Fc receptor. Science 254:1785–1788

Okazawa H, Motegi S, Ohyama N, Ohnishi H, Tomizawa T, Kaneko Y, Oldenborg PA, Ishikawa O, Matozaki T (2005) Negative regulation of phagocytosis in macrophages by the CD47-SHPS-1 system. J Immunol 174:2004–2011

Oldenborg PA, Gresham HD, Lindberg FP (2001) CD47-signal regulatory protein alpha (SIRPalpha) regulates Fcγ and complement receptor-mediated phagocytosis. J Exp Med 193:855–862

Ono M, Bolland S, Tempst P, Ravetch JV (1996) Role of the inositol phosphatase SHIP in negative regulation of the immune system by the receptor Fc(γ)RIIB. Nature 383:263–266

Ono M, Okada H, Bolland S, Yanagi S, Kurosaki T, Ravetch JV (1997) Deletion of SHIP or SHP-1 reveals two distinct pathways for inhibitory signaling. Cell 90:293–301

Otten MA, Rudolph E, Dechant M, Tuk CW, Reijmers RM, Beelen RH, van de Winkel JG, van Egmond M (2005) Immature neutrophils mediate tumor cell killing via IgA but not IgG Fc receptors. J Immunol 174:5472–5480

Padigel UM, Farrell JP (2005) Control of infection with Leishmania major in susceptible BALB/c mice lacking the common γ-chain for FcR is associated with reduced production of IL-10 and TGF-beta by parasitized cells. J Immunol 174:6340–6345

Park H, Cox D (2009) Cdc42 regulates Fc γ receptor-mediated phagocytosis through the activation and phosphorylation of Wiskott-Aldrich syndrome protein (WASP) and neural-WASP. Mol Biol Cell 20:4500–4508

Pavlou S, Wang L, Xu H, Chen M (2017) Higher phagocytic activity of thioglycollate-elicited peritoneal macrophages is related to metabolic status of the cells. J Inflamm (Lond) 14:4

Pearse RN, Kawabe T, Bolland S, Guinamard R, Kurosaki T, Ravetch JV (1999) SHIP recruitment attenuates Fc γ RIIB-induced B cell apoptosis. Immunity 10:753–760

Pegram HJ, Andrews DM, Smyth MJ, Darcy PK, Kershaw MH (2011) Activating and inhibitory receptors of natural killer cells. Immunol Cell Biol 89:216–224

Pignata C, Prasad KV, Robertson MJ, Levine H, Rudd CE, Ritz J (1993) Fc γ RIIIA-mediated signaling involves src-family lck in human natural killer cells. J Immunol 151:6794–6800

Pincetic A, Bournazos S, Dilillo DJ, Maamary J, Wang TT, Dahan R, Fiebiger BM, Ravetch JV (2014) Type I and type II Fc receptors regulate innate and adaptive immunity. Nat Immunol 15:707–716

Plotkin SA (2010) Correlates of protection induced by vaccination. Clin Vaccine Immunol 17:1055–1065

Pollara J, Easterhoff D, Fouda GG (2017) Lessons learned from human HIV vaccine trials. Curr Opin HIV AIDS 12:216–221

Pricop L, Redecha P, Teillaud JL, Frey J, Fridman WH, Sautes-Fridman C, Salmon JE (2001) Differential modulation of stimulatory and inhibitory Fc γ receptors on human monocytes by Th1 and Th2 cytokines. J Immunol 166:531–537

Qin D, Wu J, Vora KA, Ravetch JV, Szakal AK, Manser T, Tew JG (2000) Fc γ receptor IIB on follicular dendritic cells regulates the B cell recall response. J Immunol 164:6268–6275

Rakebrandt N, Lentes S, Neumann H, James LC, Neumann-Staubitz P (2014) Antibody- and TRIM21-dependent intracellular restriction of *Salmonella enterica*. Pathog Dis 72:131–137

Regnault A, Lankar D, Lacabanne V, Rodriguez A, Thery C, Rescigno M, Saito T, Verbeek S, Bonnerot C, Ricciardi-Castagnoli P, Amigorena S (1999) Fcγ receptor-mediated induction of dendritic cell maturation and major histocompatibility complex class I-restricted antigen presentation after immune complex internalization. J Exp Med 189:371–380

Reymond A, Meroni G, Fantozzi A, Merla G, Cairo S, Luzi L, Riganelli D, Zanaria E, Messali S, Cainarca S, Guffanti A, Minucci S, Pelicci PG, Ballabio A (2001) The tripartite motif family identifies cell compartments. EMBO J 20:2140–2151

Rodriguez ME, Hellwig SM, Hozbor DF, Leusen J, van der Pol WL, van de Winkel JG (2001) Fc receptor-mediated immunity against *Bordetella pertussis*. J Immunol 167:6545–6551

Sanford JE, Lupan DM, Schlageter AM, Kozel TR (1990) Passive immunization against Cryptococcus neoformans with an isotype-switch family of monoclonal antibodies reactive with cryptococcal polysaccharide. Infect Immun 58:1919–1923

Schlageter AM, Kozel TR (1990) Opsonization of *Cryptococcus* neoformans by a family of isotype-switch variant antibodies specific for the capsular polysaccharide. Infect Immun 58:1914–1918

Schlesinger JJ, Foltzer M, Chapman S (1993) The Fc portion of antibody to yellow fever virus NS1 is a determinant of protection against YF encephalitis in mice. Virology 192:132–141

Slifka MK, Antia R, Whitmire JK, Ahmed R (1998) Humoral immunity due to long-lived plasma cells. Immunity 8:363–372

Smith P, Dilillo DJ, Bournazos S, Li F, Ravetch JV (2012) Mouse model recapitulating human Fcγ receptor structural and functional diversity. Proc Natl Acad Sci U S A 109:6181–6186

Sondermann P, Pincetic A, Maamary J, Lammens K, Ravetch JV (2013) General mechanism for modulating immunoglobulin effector function. Proc Natl Acad Sci U S A 110:9868–9872

Steevels TA, Meyaard L (2011) Immune inhibitory receptors: essential regulators of phagocyte function. Eur J Immunol 41:575–587

Stone KD, Prussin C, Metcalfe DD (2010) IgE, mast cells, basophils, and eosinophils. J Allergy Clin Immunol 125:S73–S80

Suh CI, Stull ND, Li XJ, Tian W, Price MO, Grinstein S, Yaffe MB, Atkinson S, Dinauer MC (2006) The phosphoinositide-binding protein p40phox activates the NADPH oxidase during FcγIIA receptor-induced phagocytosis. J Exp Med 203:1915–1925

Swanson JA, Hoppe AD (2004) The coordination of signaling during Fc receptor-mediated phagocytosis. J Leukoc Biol 76:1093–1103

te Velde AA, de Waal Malefijt, RENE, Huijbens RJ, De Vries, JE, Figdor CG (1992) IL-10 stimulates monocyte FcγR surface expression and cytotoxic activity. Distinct regulation of antibody-dependent cellular cytotoxicity by IFN-γ, IL-4, and IL-10. J Immunol 149(12):4048–4052

Tecchio C, Micheletti A, Cassatella MA (2014) Neutrophil-derived cytokines: facts beyond expression. Front Immunol 5:508

Theofilopoulos AN, Andrews BS, Urist MM, Morton DL, Dixon FJ (1977) The nature of immune complexes in human cancer sera. J Immunol 119:657–663

Tian H, Weber S, Thorkildson P, Kozel TR, Pirofski LA (2009) Efficacy of opsonic and nonopsonic serotype 3 pneumococcal capsular polysaccharide-specific monoclonal antibodies against intranasal challenge with *Streptococcus pneumoniae* in mice. Infect Immun 77:1502–1513

Tobar JA, Gonzalez PA, Kalergis AM (2004) Salmonella escape from antigen presentation can be overcome by targeting bacteria to Fc γ receptors on dendritic cells. J Immunol 173:4058–4065

Tsai JF, Margolis HS, Jeng JE, Ho MS, Chang WY, Lin ZY, Tsai JH (1995) Circulating immune complexes in chronic hepatitis related to hepatitis C and B viruses infection. Clin Immunol Immunopathol 75:39–44

Uciechowski P, Schwarz M, Gessner JE, Schmidt RE, Resch K, Radeke HH (1998) IFN-γ induces the high-affinity Fc receptor I for IgG (CD64) on human glomerular mesangial cells. Eur J Immunol 28:2928–2935

Varshney AK, Wang X, Aguilar JL, Scharff MD, Fries BC (2014) Isotype switching increases efficacy of antibody protection against staphylococcal enterotoxin B-induced lethal shock and *Staphylococcus aureus* sepsis in mice. MBio 5:e01007–e01014

Varshney AK, Wang X, Cook E, Dutta K, Scharff MD, Goger MJ, Fries BC (2011) Generation, characterization, and epitope mapping of neutralizing and protective monoclonal antibodies against staphylococcal enterotoxin B-induced lethal shock. J Biol Chem 286:9737–9747

Varshney AK, Wang X, Scharff MD, Macintyre J, Zollner RS, Kovalenko OV, Martinez LR, Byrne FR, Fries BC (2013) Staphylococcal Enterotoxin B-specific monoclonal antibody 20B1 successfully treats diverse *Staphylococcus aureus* infections. J Infect Dis 208:2058–2066

Verma A, Ngundi MM, Meade BD, de Pascalis R, Elkins KL, Burns DL (2009) Analysis of the Fc γ receptor-dependent component of neutralization measured by anthrax toxin neutralization assays. Clin Vaccine Immunol 16:1405–1412

Von Pawel-Rammingen U, Johansson BP, Bjorck L (2002) IdeS, a novel streptococcal cysteine proteinase with unique specificity for immunoglobulin G. EMBO J 21:1607–1615

Voskoboinik I, Whisstock JC, Trapani JA (2015) Perforin and granzymes: function, dysfunction and human pathology. Nat Rev Immunol 15:388–400

Wang TT, Maamary J, Tan GS, Bournazos S, Davis CW, Krammer F, Schlesinger SJ, Palese P, Ahmed R, Ravetch JV (2015) Anti-HA glycoforms drive B cell affinity selection and determine influenza vaccine efficacy. Cell 162:160–169

Weber S, Tian H, van Rooijen N, Pirofski LA (2012) A serotype 3 pneumococcal capsular polysaccharide-specific monoclonal antibody requires Fcγ receptor III and macrophages to mediate protection against pneumococcal pneumonia in mice. Infect Immun 80:1314–1322

Weber SS, Ducry J, Oxenius A (2014) Dissecting the contribution of IgG subclasses in restricting airway infection with *Legionella pneumophila*. J Immunol 193:4053–4059

Wieland A, Kamphorst AO, Valanparambil RM, Han JH, Xu X, Choudhury BP, Ahmed R (2018) Enhancing FcγR-mediated antibody effector function during persistent viral infection. Sci Immunol 3(27):eaao3125

Wieland A, Shashidharamurthy R, Kamphorst AO, Han JH, Aubert RD, Choudhury BP, Stowell SR, Lee J, Punkosdy GA, Shlomchik MJ, Selvaraj P, Ahmed R (2015) Antibody effector functions mediated by Fcγ-receptors are compromised during persistent viral infection. Immunity 42:367–378

Woelbing F, Kostka SL, Moelle K, Belkaid Y, Sunderkoetter C, Verbeek S, Waisman A, Nigg AP, Knop J, Udey MC, von Stebut E (2006) Uptake of Leishmania major by dendritic cells is mediated by Fcγ receptors and facilitates acquisition of protective immunity. J Exp Med 203:177–188

Wrammert J, Koutsonanos D, Li GM, Edupuganti S, Sui J, Morrissey M, McCausland M, Skountzou I, Hornig M, Lipkin WI, Mehta A, Razavi B, del Rio C, Zheng NY, Lee JH, Huang M, Ali Z, Kaur K, Andrews S, Amara RR, Wang Y, Das SR, O'Donnell CD, Yewdell JW, Subbarao K, Marasco WA, Mulligan MJ, Compans R, Ahmed R, Wilson PC (2011) Broadly cross-reactive antibodies dominate the human B cell response against 2009 pandemic H1N1 influenza virus infection. J Exp Med 208:181–193

Yamada DH, Elsaesser H, Lux A, Timmerman JM, Morrison SL, de la Torre JC, Nimmerjahn F, Brooks DG (2015) Suppression of Fcγ-receptor-mediated antibody effector function during persistent viral infection. Immunity 42:379–390

Yuan R, Clynes R, Oh J, Ravetch JV, Scharff MD (1998) Antibody-mediated modulation of *Cryptococcus* neoformans infection is dependent on distinct Fc receptor functions and IgG subclasses. J Exp Med 187:641–648

Printed in the United States
By Bookmasters